THIS IS
PSYCHIATRY

Second Edition

THIS IS PSYCHIATRY

FELIX VON MENDELSSOHN, M.D.

Formerly Assistant Clinical Director,
National Institute of Mental Health, and
Associate Clinical Professor of Psychiatry,
Georgetown University, Washington, D. C.

Intercontinental Medical Book Corporation   *New York*

First Edition copyright © 1964
Franklin Watts, Inc.
Rights released to Felix von Mendelssohn, M.D., 1970

Second Edition copyright © 1973
Intercontinental Medical Book Corporation
381 Park Avenue South
New York, N. Y. 10016

Library of Congress Catalog Card No. 72-14443
ISBN 0-913258-07-5

Printed in U. S. A.

Contents

*Those medical books, those monuments
of nature's frailty and art's might! When
they tell us about the least significant
malady they make us tremble for fear of
death, but once they speak about the vir-
tue of their remedies, they bask us in
heavenly security, as if already we had
become immortal.*

MONTESQUIEU

Preface to the Second Edition

Since the original publication of this book under the title "This Is Psychiatry," Franklin Watts, Inc., New York, 1964, no decisive changes in theory or practice of psychiatry have taken place. As could be expected, more or less, both have followed the path of progress the author visualized in the first edition. Taking account of this development and progress, appropriate corrections and additions have been made, particularly in the chapters on etiology and biochemistry of the schizophrenias and manic-depressive disorders. Research in these areas continues to be intense and concerns all major sectors, i.e., genetics, brain physiology, psychological development, interactions and modes of communication within the families of patients, and sociological conditions favoring the emergence of these and other emotional disorders.

With regard to therapy, the development of the community mental health centers has continued, although not as smoothly and rapidly as one would have hoped. Much rethinking as to their philosophy, organization and staffing is in progress. Also, financial support has fallen short of expectation.

The total number of residents at any given time in State Mental Hospitals has further declined, with a simultaneous increase in first and second admissions. This is reflected in the updated statistics in the chapter on Mental Health in the United States.

More general hospitals have established small psychiatric wards and emergency treatment facilities, and there an ever increasing proportion of patients are being cared for.

Also as expected, new psychoeffective drugs have become available, mostly as chemical variations of the older ones. Lithium carbonate is now being widely accepted as the drug of choice for the manic phases of manic-depressive disorders.

In the field of psychotherapy, interest in pure and orthodox psychoanalysis has further declined and generally the approach in research and practice in this field has become a more comprehensive one, including data from research in other areas. Behavioral and conditioning therapies are being refined and more frequently applied, and so are group-therapy, family-therapy and the more controversial sessions of sensitivity training.

Last but not least, insurance companies are discovering that mental disorders are not such hopeless causes after all, and many of the companies have started to cover treatment for the mentally ill.

All these are steps in the right direction, but much remains to be done and nothing would be further from the truth than that present research in the field of mental health and illness offers any reasons for complacency. Although many older theories and concepts are being challenged and some have been put to rest, comprehensive theories and causative treatment modalities, particularly with respect to our two major problems, the schizophrenias and manic-depressive disorders, are still sadly lacking.

Finally, to this edition has been added a brief chapter on the basic principles of forensic psychiatry.

Preface to the First Edition

Today, mental health and illness are being discussed more frequently and more openly than ever before. There is a growing awareness of the existence and the manifold consequences of mental disorders. Personnel management recognizes the negative influence of emotional disturbance on industrial production. The high rejection rate of draftees during the last World War and the still considerable number of discharges of soldiers from active service on account of mental imbalance are disturbing facts. To the satisfaction of many and the chagrin of some, psychiatry has taken a front seat in the Courts of Justice. It has entered the living room through the television screen and, last but not least, mental illness and mental retardation have become a serious and acute concern for federal, state, and local legislatures.

Psychiatry, rooted in biology and reaching out into the spiritual, involves that particular part of the body, the brain, whose proper functioning we are most sensitive about. Our knowledge in psychiatric matters remains incomplete and there is an abundance of seemingly contradictory theories. These may be some of the reasons why it happens that in discussing problems of mental illness, otherwise quiet and reasonable people quickly become emotionally involved and hence unreasonable. Psychiatry, it seems, possesses all the ingredients for inviting bias and creating self-styled experts.

The aim of this book is to provide guidance through the easily confusing maze that constitutes modern psychiatry. It is dedicated to those who, while not psychiatrists, are nevertheless frequently faced in their professional lives with problems of emotional disturbance. It also addresses itself to those many others genuinely interested in psychiatry but unwilling or unable to avail themselves of the lengthy textbooks written in the idiom of the initiated.

Although the reader will find a description of the essential symptoms of different illnesses, the emphasis will be placed on an attempt to convey basic concepts and principles of psychiatry, a frame of reference for the understanding of mental illness, its causes, symptoms, and treatment.

The author will make every effort to be short and concise in his exposition, yet he will endeavor neither to sacrifice truth for the sake of "clarity" nor to dress up ignorance or unpleasant facts for the sake of a "good story."

Presently, there exist a variety of theoretical viewpoints from which mental illness is being investigated.

There are divided opinions and uncertainties as to how man develops, physiologically as well as psychologically; what, philosophically speaking, his goal or purpose is, and how he may fail in life and become mentally ill.

The title of this book is not intended to convey the impression that the author believes himself to possess the ultimate truth in psychiatry. He will present his own viewpoint and, hopefully, state fairly in what respects he differs from the opinions of others. The author believes that a discussion of psychiatric problems should be candid as well as cautious. There is much we do know and more we do not know. We still have to listen and observe first, and when we formulate theories and interpretations, we will consider them not as comfortable resting places, but as stimulants and chɔllenges on our way to finding truth.

Occasionally there is an unhappy tendency to distinguish between psychiatrists who supposedly believe only in organic or physiologic causes of mental diseases and those who place all the emphasis on psychological events as causes of mental illness. Experienced psychiatrists have never subscribed to such extreme opinions, either in the past or in our own time. Modern research in all areas pertaining to psychiatry clearly shows that the field is much too complex to allow for such primitive distinctions.

After serious consideration, the author has decided not to include a section on psychiatry and the law in this book. His main reasons are as follows.

The laws concerning insanity vary greatly from state to state in America and from country to country in the rest of the world. These laws and the principles underlying them are currently undergoing radical changes, although they remain as controversial as ever.

The principal issues involved concern the legal and criminal responsibility of the mentally ill and the laws governing the commitment of such individuals to institutions. When discussing these matters, the lawyer and the psychiatrist often seem to be speaking in different languages, but we hope that a better understanding will be achieved in the future.

The author hopes that the reader will obtain a sufficiently clear picture of mental illness and the mentally ill to be able to follow the legal and psychiatric arguments as they are advanced in the courts and the news media. But for a more detailed study of these problems, the reader should consult books on forensic psychiatry.

The author believes that only a truly multidimensional approach can do justice to the intricate problems of psychiatry in general and to the individual patient in particular. In this, he believes that he is following the best of European and American traditions in psychiatry. Thus, in his attitude as well as in his writings, he will try always to maintain a healthy balance between qualified doubt and justified optimism.

·I·

Historical Review

Dark Ages for Psychiatry:

PSYCHIATRY is the branch of medicine concerning itself with the study and care of mental illness. Or,
somewhat less tersely, "Psychiatry is that branch of
medicine in which psychological phenomena are important
as causes, signs and symptoms, or as curative agents."
(Mayer-Gross, Slater and Roth)

The fact that psychiatry is a branch of medicine needs
emphasis. This is sometimes overlooked. It should be
noted that the definition does not include as pertinent to
psychiatry the interpretation of art, the providing of goals
for the bored, nor the pronouncement of sweeping

1

statements on the character of entire nations. A psychiatrist is a physician, not a missionary. Occasional misunderstandings in this respect do occur.

Psychiatry has not always been a branch of medicine and the mentally ill have not always been cared for by physicians. A glance at history will quickly show what it has meant at various times to be mentally ill.

Through the ages the mentally ill have puzzled, mystified, and, more than anything else, frightened their fellow-men, who have tried to understand and control them in accordance with the beliefs and mores of the time. Beliefs and mores have not always been kind to the mentally ill.

In ancient Greece, a few physicians realized that mental illness was not a curse from a god, but a disease as natural as pneumonia. Such notions did not survive long. Throughout most of the following centuries, the mentally ill person was believed to be possessed by evil spirits and his fate remained in the hands of the priest. It seems fair to assume that many mentally ill died on the stakes of the Inquisition. Others, who resisted exorcism and survived torture, were likely to be kept in jails and dungeons, often chained to the wall.

In the fifteenth century, hope was kindled when Johann Weyer, a German physician, once more taught that mental illness was medical illness and should be treated by physicians. His books were banned by the Church, but here and there his thoughts had fallen on fertile ground. In the eighteenth and nineteenth centuries, though tremendous progress occurred in all sciences, including the medical sciences, psychiatry profited relatively little. Only gradually and hesitatingly did the concern with the mind and its distortions slip from the province of the priest and the philosopher into that of the physician, who also often tried hard to be a philosopher and moralist first.

Clinical Observations and Moral Treatment:

Changes began to take place after the French Revolution. Kind and keen physicians improved the lot of mental patients and began to assemble an impressive body of careful clinical observations. Such men were Philippe Pinel and Jean Esquirol in France, Griesinger in Germany, Henry Maudsley in England, and Benjamin Rush and Isaac Ray in the United States. New hospitals were built, case histories and occasional statistics were kept. Great efforts were made to rebuild the patient's self-esteem and dignity through what became known as "moral treatment." Hospitals were small and the patients were treated like members of a large family gathered around a paternal superintendent who ate with them and shared many of their activities, always setting an example of normal living. Yet theories concerning the causes of mental illness remained frequently bizarre. An admixture of religious and moral ideas with poorly understood medical concepts accounted for the fact that specific treatment remained mostly crude, intentionally punitive, frightening, and painful. Rotating chairs, sudden and unsuspected showers of cold water, ghost chambers, and, of course, extensive bloodletting were some of the therapeutic measures in use until late in the nineteenth century.

In contrast to this period of idealistic reorientation and gathering of clinical observations, the decades of the outgoing nineteenth and the beginning twentieth century became a time of crystallization of theories and classification of mental diseases.

The Quest for Order and Understanding:

Attempts to bring order into the often confusing symptomatology of mental illness had been made at various times. Yet, at the middle of the last century there was no generally accepted classification of mental diseases. The natural sciences, and hence logical causative thinking, dominated the scene, and physicians, in general, followed this trend. But in psychiatry, just emerging as a separate discipline of medicine, little was known about the causes of the symptom clusters which seemed to constitute distinctive diseases. Causes were sought for primarily within the brain, and so neurologists and pathologists, equipped with the microscope, started to play a leading role in psychiatric research. Such symptoms as mental confusion, forgetfulness, and erratic behavior in the aged were correlated with degenerative changes observable in the brain itself. In some chronic alcoholics, symptoms of physical, as well as mental, deterioration could be linked to the destruction by alcohol of specific parts of the brain. At the same time, it occasionally appeared justifiable to link some symptoms of mental stress to specific traumatic events in a patient's emotional life. Thus, an emotional depression could be attributed to the loss of a loved one, if the first immediately followed the latter. But there remained a great number of mental patients whose disorders did not fit into either one of these categories of causation.

The only logical alternative was to classify these disorders according to their observable symptoms or symptom clusters and their overall course. It became clear, for example, that certain symptom complexes tended to appear early in life and led more or less regularly to progressive mental deterioration. Symptoms of a different type would emerge at a later stage in life and disappear again, with a tendency to recur. Such criteria and others, which will be discussed later, finally led to a classification of mental disorders that still serves as a basic frame of reference for almost all official modern classifications.

The two men primarily responsible for this historical work were Emil Kraepelin in Germany and Eugen Bleuler in Switzerland. They were truly great observers, forever revising their own work, and well realizing that due to the lack of etiological knowledge, their classification could not be final.

While Kraepelin and Bleuler were putting order into their data, Ivan P. Pavlov, a Russian physiologist, conducted animal experiments to study what he called unlearned (or unconditioned) and learned (or conditioned) reflexes. For example, he had observed that a dog begins to salivate as soon as it sees its food. This represents an unconditioned reflex. But if for a certain period a bell rings at the same time the food is being offered, the dog will finally salivate at the sound of the bell alone, without seeing the food. Thus, a new reflex has been conditioned. The disruption of the newly established reflex by sudden and irregular changes in the bell ringing and food serving will then produce in the dog behavior marked by confusion, anxiety, nervousness, and refusal to eat. Such symptoms were believed to be comparable to symptoms in some mental disorders, and it was hypothesized that much, if not all, of man's normal and abnormal behavior is based on unconditioned and conditioned reflexes.

A great amount of work has been conducted along these lines and much of the official modern psychiatry in Russia is based on Pavlov's ideas. Based on these learning theories a system of psychotherapeutic techniques, under the name of behavioral therapy, is presently gaining increasing recognition. Although there are many fascinating aspects to these theories, experiments and practical applications, it is too early for us to assess all their theoretic and therapeutic implications.

It remains for us to mention yet another approach in the struggle toward the understanding of mental illness. This is the attempt to conceive of mental disorders as the result of intimate emotional experiences, of cultural patterns, and environmental circumstances. The foundations of this field of research, which is presently rather prominent, were also consolidated during the latter part of the last century.

Man has always sought to comprehend himself, to understand his own emotional development, behavior, and purpose in religious and philosophic terms. It seemed only natural to include in such speculations the unusual behavior and experiences of the mentally ill. Thus, many psychiatrists remained unsatisfied with the mere description of symptoms of mental disorders and the use of them as diagnostic criteria. What these men hoped to find was the secret behind the symptom, the key to the meaning of the bizarre behavior. Hypnosis, at the time much experimented with in France, seemed to be a suitable method to reach this goal. Under hypnosis, a person would have peculiar sensations and show strange behavior as suggested to him. Hypnosis also promised to divulge some of the key secrets of the emotionally disturbed person. Later, other methods were established which seemed to permit the establishment of meaningful connections between experiences in the patient's life and symptoms of emotional disorders. Gradually some psychiatrists came to regard a symptom, a sequence of symptoms, or, more generally, abnormal behavior and sensations as a patient's particular way of avoiding or fighting emotional stress.

For example, a young woman may complain of sudden blindness for which physical examination finds no explanation. Intensive interviews reveal that the emotionally unstable patient has just maneuvered herself into a difficult and unpleasant situation with a married man, involving a quick decision on her part as to what to do next. The blindness, appearing at this critical moment, could be conceived of as being a symbolic expression of the patient's fear and unwillingness to see and face the situation at hand. The patient herself remains unaware or unconscious of the true motivation and the nature of the blindness. The disappearance of the symptom after an acceptable solution to the girl's situation has been found would in this particular case support the evidence of a cause and effect sequence between emotional stress and symptom.

In organizing the apparent knowledge gathered on the basis of such concepts, different theories were formulated with regard to man's psychic development and the nature of his emotional disorders. As yet, there is little similarity or agreement among these theories. They tend to emphasize as decisive in the development of emotional distortions, rather different aspects of man's life, such as his sexual drives, his need for power and superiority, or his aspirations for spiritual fulfillment. However, all such theories have in common two major aspects which are important to remember. They contain teleological, or goal-directed, concepts as to man's purpose in life, and their key element is the unconscious.

If this tends to limit their scientific or explanatory value with regard to causation in mental disorders, they have nevertheless decisively stimulated modern psychiatry. Whatever the final judgment may be as to their theoretical concepts, we do believe that the outstanding men in this field, such as Pierre Janet in France, Sigmund Freud and Alfred Adler in Austria, Carl G. Jung and Ludwig Binswanger in Switzerland, have made lasting contributions to the understanding of man's behavior in general, and of the mentally ill in particular. Some of their basic concepts have subsequently been altered, adjusted, and expanded in various ways. They have stimulated research in many areas pertaining to man's environment and circumstances that may contribute to mental disorders. The principal tenets of modern psychotherapy rest on their work.

Advances in Treatment:

Quite independently of all theoretical formulations and efforts to arrive at a comprehensive classification, a series of important events concerning therapy took place during the first half of our own century.

First came the successful treatment of progressive paralysis. The initial linking of the clinical symptoms of progressive mental and physical deterioration to syphilis, the following microscopic demonstration of the causative agent in the brain, the *spirochaeta pallida*, and the final arrest of the illness by elimination of the spirochaete with chemical treatment have remained a classical example of scientific procedure in medicine. For psychiatry, so far, this is the only specific therapy for a major mental illness. Once, the patient with progressive paralysis was one of the principal long-term occupants of mental hospitals. Today, due to the early and successful treatment of syphilis with penicillin, hospital admission of such a patient is rare in Europe and in the United States.

Other therapeutic methods were discovered rather accidentally and developed empirically. We will only mention them briefly here because they will be dealt with in more detail in the chapter on therapy.

In 1933, M. J. Sakel, in Austria, introduced insulin coma therapy for the treatment of schizophrenia. In 1935, L. J. Meduna observed that schizophrenic patients seemed to get better as far as their schizophrenic symptoms were concerned when they had spontaneous epileptic seizures. Consequently, he sought methods of producing seizures artificially, and thus introduced metrazol shock therapy, which, in 1938, was replaced with electroshock therapy by U. Cerletti and L. Bini in Italy.

In 1936, A. Egaz Moniz, in Portugal, demonstrated that frontal lobotomy, a surgical separation of certain nerve tracts within the brain, could alleviate severe anxiety and other disturbing mental symptoms.

In 1952, J. Delay and P. Denniker, in France, opened up an entirely new area in the treatment of mental patients. They discovered and introduced chlorpromazine (Thorazine), the first of a long series of chemical agents with peculiar tranquilizing effects on mental patients.

One of these drugs, while in the experimental stage, was discovered by R. Kuhn in Switzerland to have activating effects in depressed patients rather than the intended tranquilizing of agitated schizophrenics. This drug, now known as Tofranil, has remained one of the most potent of a series of antidepressant drugs developed since 1953.

The ultimate value of all these "psychoeffective" (F. A. Freyhan) drugs remains an open question. However, there can be no doubt that they have radically changed the lives of many patients, and the atmosphere of mental hospitals. Gone are the straitjackets, the mechanical restraints, most of the isolation rooms, and the noisy and turbulent day-rooms. Today, in psychiatric wards, we find pictures on the walls, plants and vases on tables, patients sitting or ambulating quietly, engaged in various activities. Many of the previously locked doors are open and patients come and go.

Not all of this must or can be attributed to the effectiveness of these drugs, and in many instances what we see are chain reactions. We may consider, for instance, fifty chronic mental patients sitting or lying around on benches in a rather dark, poorly ventilated, overcrowded ward. They have been there doing nothing for a number of years. Nurses and nursing assistants have despaired. A young physician who must take care of four hundred other patients visits briefly once a day. At this point, a new therapeutic agent such as a psychoeffective drug is introduced and proves helpful in approximately ten patients. These ten suddenly become more active, rational, and interested. One of them may be transferred to a better ward. When this is observed by the other patients it may mean to some that there is hope, and they, in turn, will become more lively and active. The physician and the nursing personnel become stimulated and enthusiastic. Someone realizes that the ward is dark and dirty and needs painting. New activities are started for more and more patients. Some of them improve moderately, some greatly, and some may even be able to leave the hospital. In such a chain reaction it is difficult to decide what can be attributed to drug effect and what to other factors, the most important of which may well be the moral climate of the ward.

Finally, brief mention must be made of the gradual emergence during the past 50 years of psychotherapy as an independent and well-developed therapeutic tool. Psychotherapy, or psychological treatment, of course has always existed in one form or another. It was utilized by the priests of ancient Egypt and Greece, by the witch doctor in Africa, and by physicians in all centuries.

As we indicated earlier, much of modern Western psychotherapy is based on the works of Freud (psychoanalysis), and less so on those of Adler (individual psychology), Jung (analytical psychology), and Binswanger (existential analysis). Whenever philosophy and personal inclinations enter a field of human endeavor, disagreement over principles and the foundation of different schools are the result, and psychotherapy did not escape this fate. It has developed along different lines of thought and today we are confronted with a variety of "schools." In general, original theoretical concepts have been broadened and therapeutic techniques have been revised. For some schools the area for application of psychotherapy, in one way or another, is composed of almost all forms of mental disorder. Yet the impact of psychotherapy on psychiatric illness has remained a controversial issue.

Last but not least, intensive laboratory research and sociologic studies in the field have opened new avenues to our understanding of mental illness. Brain physiology is focusing attention on certain biochemical events seemingly involved in illnesses such as schizophrenia and manic-depressive disease. Refined family studies of such patients, together with an increasing understanding of the bio-chemical structure of the genetic code, shed new light and confirmation on older empirical concepts of hereditary factors. Finally, more sophisticated research into family interaction and the psychological and sociological implica-tions of community life are refining our analytical under-standing; we group these concepts under the term, communication.

Summary:

In summarizing this necessarily incomplete historical survey, we might say that after a long journey under different flags the psychiatrist has now taken his seat as a full member in the assembly of medical specialists. Observational material has been collected and some order wrought. Yet some of the most devastating mental diseases have remained elusive in terms of causation, diagnosis, and therapy. Certainly there is no lack of theories and enthusiasm, but there is a lack of concrete knowledge. The lot of the mental patient has undoubtedly been greatly improved, particularly since the advent of modern methods of treatment. The general attitude toward the mentally ill is gradually changing, and superstition and bias are giving way to a more realistic approach.

We have entered a period of great expectations, a period of intense theoretical and practical activity and research, a period in which much of the thinking in psychiatry is in constant flux. To those who see the still unsolved problems, the study and treatment of the mentally ill remains one of the great challenges of our time.

·II·

Concepts of Mental Disorders

Definition:

PROPERLY, a book on mental disorders should begin with definitions of such terms as mental or emotional disorders or mental illness. Yet this is not easily done, nor is it certain that a discussion of this question would be enlightening or fruitful. There is no uniform definition of illness even in strictly somatic medicine, let alone in psychiatry.

As a manifestation of the brain, mental illness is rooted in biology but it is also the result of constant interaction between the brain and the environment with all its social, cultural, and religious implications. We can expect constancy in the first and change in the latter. The most pragmatic definition might be a social one, but we cannot use the same measure throughout. Psychiatry is in transition; some of its aspects we know well at the level of scientific knowledge, others we merely suspect, and many are simply unknown.

Taking a first step in defining our topic one can say this: the mentally abnormal person is one who experiences, feels, thinks or acts in a way that sets him apart from the average population around him. But this is a mere description and not a definition. Also, we must be mindful that the borders between health and illness are not clearly marked, neither in somatic medicine nor in psychiatry.

Over a century ago W. Griesinger in Germany declared that all mental disorders are disorders of the brain, meaning that all must have a biological basis. If this were true, we would have an ideal definition, but in the light of our present knowledge this theory, which dominated psychiatry for a long time, cannot be upheld. On the opposite side we hear some say that mental illness does not really exist at all, is a myth, the psychological product of a mismanaged society. Such gratuitous statements do not seem to be well founded in clinical experience and are presented with often vexing pseudo-logical arguments. They share many of the fallacies that mark psychological and sociological definitions of mental health and illness. Thus, by saying that mental health is a state of total well-being, of maximal emotional growth and happiness, of the ability to adjust and so forth, and mental illness the opposite or lack of all this, not much is being said at all. Such statements are too vague and subjective to be useful. Also, if we were to assume that the standard of normalcy is to be set by the prevailing forces in a given society we will quickly find ourselves on very slippery ground. We will be forced to operate with such questionable concepts as "average" and "adjustment to the average" and will soon lose all scientific credentials. Neither is it the task of the psychiatrist to define how the average population ought to think and act, nor is he bound to accept the average population's thoughts and actions as his yardstick for health and illness.

Actually, because of many factors as yet unknown we are simply not in a position to present an all-embracing, unifying definition of mental illness. However, if we are more modest, we can come closer to it. The author shares the opinion of those who hold that in defining the field of psychiatry we must adhere to what has been called the medical model. Medicine must remain the basis for our operation. By the same token we must realize and admit that this medical model embraces medical as well as psychological and to a much lesser degree sociological concepts. Thus, we revert to the scientifically more reliable medico-psychological concepts of individual mental functions and their aberrations.

These mental functions are threefold: firstly, they concern *cognition,* or what in a later chapter we call input. Here we consider visual, auditory, tactile, gustatory and olfactory perceptions, in other words the five senses. Secondly, we summarize under the term *affect* such modalities as mood and sensitivity. Thirdly, *conation* pertains to thinking and motivation resulting in outward behavior, or what we have termed output. Aberrations in these functions can be traced in all mental disorders, from abnormal reactions to organic brain syndromes, as will be

Taste   Hear
Smell
Feel
See

seen in subsequent chapters. Thus, these concepts provide us with certain common denominators.

Finally, we can add the three traditional medical criteria which will help us to recognize mental illness:

1. The patient feels ill, which is a general subjective datum. (However, some patently psychotic patients, like the paranoid schizophrenic or the manic, will not readily admit to being ill.)

2. The patient has disordered function of some part of him, which is a restricted objective datum.

3. He has symptoms which conform to a recognizable clinical pattern, which is a typological datum. (Sir Aubrey Lewis: "Health as a social concept," in *The State of Psychiatry*, Science Books, New York, 1967, p. 187.)

With these criteria in mind we will now proceed in our attempt to further define our subject and draw some lines separating major groups of mental disorders. The first group primarily contains the neuroses and character disorders. By definition, these show signs and symptoms which differ quantitatively but not qualitatively from normal feeling, thinking, and behaving. For instance, hallucinations, delusions, or disorientation in time and place are never part of such disorders. Thus, we define them as abnormal variations of normal human behavior.

In the second group we find mental disorders that result from, or are part of, known somatic diseases. Here we include psychic symptoms due to brain damage and toxic or infectious conditions.

The third and final group consists of the two most important but so far equally elusive psychiatric entities, schizophrenia and manic-depressive disease. As to their etiology, nothing definite can be stated at the time of this writing.

In this book, the terms emotional or mental disorder, illness or disease, will be used interchangeably. The term psychosis is used differently in the United States from the way it is used in Europe. In the United States, it is frequently used pragmatically and quantitatively, denoting the degree of severity of an illness. A person is psychotic if he has lost contact with reality, whether on account of delusions or loss of orientation. Thus, an individual can be schizophrenic with symptoms so mild that he is in contact with reality and consequently is not psychotic. In much of European psychiatry the term has qualitative connotations and, by definition, pertains to all disorders of our groups two and three but not to those of group one. Accordingly, a schizophrenic patient is psychotic no matter how few symptoms he may show, and a neurotic person is not psychotic however handicapped he may be by his neurosis.

Psychic Functions Impaired in Mental Disorders:

Although the size and structure of this book do not permit extensive discussion of the psychology and physiology of normal human development and behavior, it is necessary to mention briefly some of the basic psychological functions that can be disturbed in mental illness. In so doing we will borrow from the language and concepts of the information theory and the electronic computer sciences.

The brain is the central organ where external stimuli from man's environment and internal stimuli from within his own body are received and evaluated and where action is determined. From the brain, messages are sent back to the world and the body as reactions and seemingly spontaneous actions. Thus in many ways the brain resembles an electronic computer which, after having been fed such information as figures for multiplication, produces a written answer. The impulses, information, or messages that reach the brain can be called input, and those that leave it, output. To input belong visual and auditory, gustatory and tactile impressions, i.e., impressions of things we see, hear, taste, and feel. To output belong activities such as closing the eyes, speaking, smiling, scratching, or walking. Both external stimuli and reactions through muscles reach and leave the brain primarily through a system of sensory and motor nerves. To the brain the vegetative nervous system sends stimuli originating in internal organs like the stomach and heart, and brings regulative orders back to them leading, for instance, to the excretion of stomach juice or the slowing of the heartbeat.

The most complex and mysterious part of this input and output system is the operation of the brain itself in correlating, evaluating and storing information and transforming it into action.

Modern physiology teaches that these various functions are not localized but that more or less the entire brain is involved in each cerebral transaction. An intricate system of checks and balances, of transcerebral connections in which electrical, hormonal and other chemical reactions influence each other, forms the basic structure for all that connects input with output or reaction. Drive, affectivity and intellect are the particularly human elements missing in computers, that permeate, color, and influence all these processes.

The way these processes function and how they can be disturbed by mental illness is best demonstrated by an example. Let us choose the one forever young and classic: boy sees girl.

First the image of the girl registers on the retina of the young man. The image, in the form of electrical impulses, is relayed from the eye along the optic nerve and optic tract to very specific areas of the brain, terminating at its posterior pole. The various relay stations through which it passes are connected with, controlled by, and in turn control many other structures throughout the brain. Whether or not the image of the girl is perceived clearly or dimly, or is permitted to reach the brain at all, is controlled through fine nerve fibers traveling along the optic nerve and tract, but in the opposite direction, i.e., from the brain to the eye. According to demand and readiness, these fibers regulate the input and transmission of the message.

At the posterior pole of the brain, with the help of stored memories about shapes and colors of girls, the incoming impulses are recognized as the image of a girl. Again, speed and clarity of recognition can be regulated by adjacent parts of the brain. Immediately, the emergence of the image of the girl may activate various other structures of the brain leading to the appearance of other memories about girls, and the evaluation of the girl in terms of beauty, intelligence, social status or accessibility. Sexual desires may be aroused together with thoughts of mother's disapproval. The direction in which all this is going to lead will depend on the young man's upbringing, previous experience, degree of impulsivity, mood, and other criteria.

Having sifted and weighed all this information, i.e., having debated in his mind what to do, our friend will proceed with some action: a disinterested walking away, a faint smile in the direction of the girl, a waving of the hand, or an engaging "good morning." His reaction may not be restricted to such motor actions but may include outgoing impulses through the vegetative nervous system, which increase his heartbeat, or cause sudden sweating or other bodily functions commensurate with his thoughts and feelings. However, if our friend had been absorbed in a philosophical conversation, he might not even have "seen" the girl, although her image was captured by his retina and stored away in some area of his brain.

The last sentence must focus our attention on yet another important factor in the functioning of the mind—conscious and unconscious psychic processes. Our friend, whom we will call Benjamin, could have stored the image of the girl without even knowing about it. This would have been an unconscious process. Once stored, the image would have become part of Benjamin's memory, and as such it could be recalled or made conscious at a later date. Furthermore, when we mentioned thoughts, ideas and doubts that crossed Benjamin's mind, it was with the understanding that he was conscious of them when he decided to act. Had Benjamin been less deliberate, or conscious, he might have acted instantaneously in one way or another without realizing what prompted his action. This would have been an unconscious reaction.

It is widely assumed that the majority of man's motivations and desires are unconscious. Some of them are brought to consciousness at will and when needed, others only with the help of analysis or hypnosis, but most remain unconscious. Much has been written and said about man's unconscious. Indeed, the exploration of the unconscious may be a desirable task. But, the inherent danger is that the unconscious defies inductive or logical scientific methods of investigation. It invites deductive thinking, starting from preconceived ideas about man's destiny and ending in speculations and fancy interpretations that can be neither proved nor disproved.

But let us return to our model. Input, intracerebral transactions and output are clearly recognizable. We might add that the entire process as described will be stored as memory, becoming unconscious but remaining on call for later reference. It will be joined by memory imprints concerning the result of Benjamin's action and the entire complex will perhaps influence our friend's future behavior in the presence of girls. In the following, we will show how, in general terms, mental disorders can distort the functions constituting the input-output system.

Diseases of the nerves that send information from the periphery to the brain and from the brain to muscles are almost invariably physical or neurological in nature. If such nerves are injured through trauma, infection, or toxic substances, the brain will receive no sensations or abnormal ones, such as numbness in the fingers or limpness in muscles, because messages to them cannot get through. (Example: poliomyelitis.) Some diseases, such as chronic alcoholism which attacks the peripheral nervous system, also affect the brain, causing psychological symptoms. Also, we encounter persons claiming numbness or weakness in an extremity. In such cases, in the absence of physical abnormalities in the areas supposedly affected, one may stipulate faulty interpretation and decision-making within the brain itself.

The realm of psychiatry is the intracerebral operation of our system and the outside repercussions of these, i.e., everything that happens from the moment a message is received until an idea is formed or a response is sent out. Incoming impulses may be ignored, overemphasized or misinterpreted. They may be connected illogically with other information, with too few or too many previous impressions. Memory may be inaccessible or lost, which makes identification of incoming messages difficult, faulty or impossible. Mood may be depressed or elated, or an all-pervasive disinterest in human relationships may prevail. Finally, enigmatic phenomena, such as illusions, delusions, and hallucinations may interfere with appropriate thinking, feeling and acting. More about this will be said in the chapters on the different mental disorders. Here, a few examples will suffice to illustrate what is meant.

In neuroses, painful memories may be kept unconscious, but they nevertheless interfere with the formation of rational decisions in certain areas. In a depressed person, the low mood and energy level are the central problems. Most psychic and some bodily functions will be slowed down, and incoming messages may be adversely misinterpreted, evoking only the worst memories. The outflow of messages will be sparse; the patient will sit and brood. In another example, an old man who has had a stroke loses much of his memory through destruction of brain tissue. Incoming information cannot be identified because corresponding memory traces are no longer available. There are misinterpretations and a general paucity of correlations and the patient feels confused and suspicious since he does not understand what is going on. Mood may be labile and outgoing messages become erratic and purposeless.

We have discussed different functions that can be disturbed in mental disorders. We have used this approach for practical and didactic reasons. Frequently one hears that the physician ought not to consider functions but rather the patient in his totality. Often, we suspect, such criticism is gratuitous and seems to stem more from lack of precise knowledge than from concern for the patient. Throughout the centuries, true physicians have tried to understand their patients and not merely their symptoms. Indeed, remarkable things have been said in this respect, and it is disconcerting to see how much knowledge has to be rediscovered over and over by successive generations. It is quite true that during the past few decades rapidly increasing knowledge in physiology, biochemistry, internal medicine, surgery, and radiology has brought about a wave of extreme medical specialization. It is more likely than not that this trend will continue as knowledge increases further. But specialization does not exclude understanding and knowledge of the connections between diseases in general and organic dysfunctions and psyche in particular. This knowledge is growing and so is the awareness of its importance. However, in theory and in therapy it would appear wiser to say or do something limited of which one is sure, than something sweeping of which one is not sure.

General Remarks on Etiology:

Blindness in one eye can have many causes. The cornea may be so opaque that no light will pass through. The lens may be diseased, and so may the visual elements of the eye ground. Further, the pathways of the visual or optic stimulation within the brain itself, the optic nerve, the optic tract, and optic radiation and visual cortex of the brain may all be the seat of lesions causing blindness. Each lesion can be caused by a variety of disorders, such as injury, infection, toxic degeneration or tumors. Blindness, then, is an unspecific symptom. Without further inquiry, one can say little about the illness causing it.

In psychiatry, there is not a single symptom which, alone and unequivocally, indicates to the physician the kind of illness that confronts him. Symptoms of mental disorders are unspecific. An auditory hallucination, a "voice," can be heard by a schizophrenic, an alcoholic in a delirium, a deeply depressed patient, and a senile person. Although there may be subtle differences in the type of voices these patients hear, the differences can give no more than a hint as to the illness involved. Both body and mind have only a limited arsenal of answers to a great number of stimuli, troubles and diseases.

Individual emotional disorders are recognized by con- stellations of symptoms—syndromes as we call them— which receive additional significance from the circum- stances under which they appear. Symptoms can shift and change and still indicate the presence of the same illness.

To illustrate this, let us take a few snapshots in a mental hospital. A girl, age twenty, sits motionless in a corner of a room, knees up to her chin, unapproachable, smiles strangely and vacantly and moves her lips in silent response to voices she alone can hear. Two days later the same girl, still responding to voices, wild-eyed and scream- ing, smashes everything she can reach. An elderly man, somewhat distant and peculiar, obviously conversing with some invisible person, cleans the washroom in the ward but takes time off to tell the visitor confidentially that, in reality, he is the Lord and owns the entire hospital. A middle-aged, undernourished, feverish-looking man, highly excited, shouting angrily in answer to voices, with trembling hands tries to remove imaginary bugs from his skin and bed.

In all three instances we see a patient responding to voices, but additional symptoms create different syndromes in each. In the girl's case, the placid mood gives way to sudden excitement, possibly in response to a different content of the voices. The second case is distinguished from the first by the age and temperament of the patient, though the man is just as much absorbed in his voices and delusions as is the girl. In both cases, the syndromes belong to the group of schizophrenias. In the last instance, the hearing of voices is embedded in a very different set of circumstances such as undernourishment, fever, restlessness, and visual and tactile hallucinations ("bugs"). The syndrome most probably indicates the presence of a toxic delirium due to excessive drinking.

In the United States, the theory has been advanced that specific mental diseases do not exist. According to this theory, symptoms and syndromes are only the psyche's gamut of defense reactions against a gamut of stressful situations. These reactions would differ from each other quantitatively but not qualitatively, as they would in the case of specific mental diseases. Thus a person would respond to mild stress with a neurotic reaction; would shift under increasing stress to a schizophrenic or psychotic reaction; and finally, under successful treatment, would revert to a neurotic one. The reader will notice that according to this theory one does not speak of illness or disease, but of "reactions" only. (If this theory were applied in internal medicine, one would call a pneumococcus pneumonia a mild reaction that eventually could lead to pulmonary tuberculosis, a severe reaction. Obviously this is absurd, since pneumococcus pneumonia and tuberculosis are two very distinct diseases.)

Such a unitary concept of mental disorders would necessarily be restricted to syndromes not due to clearly definable organic diseases. Modern research seems to indicate, however, that there are no organic diseases without psychic symptoms, and no mental disorders without physical changes. Presently, this aspect of psychiatry is in constant flux, as indicated elsewhere in this book. Moreover, experience teaches that correctly diagnosed neuroses do not develop into anything else, certainly not into anything resembling schizophrenia. To be sure, there are very serious and crippling cases of neurosis and mild ones of schizophrenia. But even in partial remission, the schizophrenic invariably remains recognizable as such. There are no transitional stages between the two conditions. Furthermore there is evidence of significant hereditary factors in schizophrenia, but there is no such evidence for neuroses. Finally, few mistakes are made in differentiating neurotics from schizophrenics, but it can be very difficult to distinguish between toxic or other organic syndromes and schizophrenia. Necessarily, in a discussion like this, one provision must be made: All participants ought to speak the same language, i.e., all should adhere, for instance, to the same official definition of schizophrenia. Much misunderstanding has resulted from private variations of this definition. But even taking the semantic problem into account, the available evidence over-whelmingly favors the acceptance of separate psychiatric diseases, although these may well have multi-factorial etiologies.

After these initial remarks about the lack of specificity of psychiatric symptoms, we will now proceed with the general considerations regarding the etiology of mental disorders.

Hereditary Factors:

Fifteen years ago, speaking about heredity and mental illness in the United States was not precisely identical with making friends. The opinion prevailed that studying heredity was an old-fashioned European pursuit, fatalistic and paralyzing to progress. The visitor could gain the impression that in the United States the acceptance of genetic etiological factors was considered incompatible with the basic American principle that men of good will should be able to change and to improve. European psychiatrists, believing in the significance of genetic factors in some mental disorders, never felt that these factors prevented therapy. After all, the shapes of skulls and feet are genetically determined, yet both were markedly altered by the Incas and the Chinese. Many arguments used confidently by the geneticists were simply turned around and used with just as much assurance by the "environ-mentalists" and vice versa. Thus, the first would consider it a matter of course that the schizophrenic mother had genetically transmitted the disease to the schizophrenic son. The latter would argue that the schizophrenic mother, cold, distant, and unable to provide motherly love, would necessarily cause the deprived son to develop schizophrenic reactions to the stresses of life. Fortunately reality is never as exclusive as theory. Research in heredity, in the United States and elsewhere, another world war and political experiences thereafter, have changed many concepts. Genetic studies have been systematized and refined and have proceeded along lines both clinical and biochemical. The results, emerging slowly, are fascinating and unexpected.

From investigating families and drawing pedigrees counting the abnormal members, genetics has largely withdrawn into the laboratories of the biochemists and microbiologists. These scientists concentrate on the most intricate and minute microscopic and chemical analyses of the structure of single cell nuclei and their individual chromosomes. It has been estimated that the 22 pairs of human chromosomes and the sex chromosomes that are present in each cell contain approximately sixty thousand genes, in the form of chemical compounds, which determine and regulate every phase of bodily growth and functions. The slightest fault or deviation in the transmission of these genes from parent to child, minimal changes in their chemical structure, or mutations will cause abnormal development or metabolic diseases. For instance, the cytogenic basis for mongolism, a form of mental deficiency, and the basis for abnormal sexual differentiation have now been firmly established. Franz J. Kallman, one of the pioneers in genetics in the U. S., who reports on this, says ". . . The list of psychiatric disorders (such as schizophrenia and manic-depressive disease identifiable as the result of gross chromosomal disarrangement will probably grow considerably within a few years . . ."*

The psychiatrist no longer thinks of a single hereditary factor striking like fate and bringing about illness. Rather, genetic factors seem to create a predisposition for a certain illness. Such a predisposition can be strong or weak, can be compensated for and checked or enhanced by other genetic or environmental forces. Thus a predisposition to schizophrenia might remain dormant in a person who was well balanced and had grown up in a secure home situation, while a similar predisposition might lead to manifest illness in another, less secure, person. There are thousands of variations possible in the interplay of different genetic endowments and the constantly changing environment, which together create what we see: a person and his fate. Genetic factors will be discussed further in the chapters on the individual disorders.

Somatotype:

One of the characteristics of man that is definitely molded by heredity is the shape of his body, or what we call his body- or somatotype. About fifty years ago the German psychiatrist Ernst Kretschmer noticed apparent relationships between certain body types and personality and mental illness. In the following decades, he and others accumulated pertinent observations and were able to define the subject with fair accuracy. In the United States, W. H. Sheldon pursued these ideas and gradually developed very accurate photographic and mathematic methods of

*Franz J. Kallman: *The Future of Psychiatry.* P. H. Hoch and J. Zubin (editors). New York, Grune & Stratton, 1962.

measuring and correlating body type, character, and illness. His research includes not only mental disorders but also other areas of general medicine.

Looking at a group of men and women on a sunny beach, one easily notices that some are rather thin, fragile, and devoid of musculature. Their heads may be small, birdlike, their necks long, their chests and abdomens lean and narrow. Their demeanor often inspires distance. On others all parts seem to be short and round. The ball-like head sits right on the barrel-shaped chest which enlarges into a well-provided abdomen. Hips are narrow. Like many round objects, these people seem to invite confidence. Finally, we recognize some whom we readily associate with ball fields and boxing rings. They are strong and solid, with massive heads, protruding lower jaws, wide chest and abdomen, and abundant musculature. Ernst Kretschmer called these body types leptosomatic, pyknic, and athletic; W. H. Sheldon named them ectomorphic, endomorphic, and mesomorphic, respectively. Both related to them rather specific personality types.

The ectomorphic tends to be a sensitive, perhaps rigid, abstract thinker and theoretician, often tense, little gregarious but apt to be tenacious in the face of opposition. He would like to change the world to suit his ideas. The endomorphic has less difficulty in accepting life as it is. More practically minded, he is jovial and relaxed but also sensitive in his emotional reactions, readily overjoyed or discouraged. The mesomorphic relies much on his physical strength. Usually a reliable and persistent worker, he holds on to what he has. His temperament has been called viscous.

Obviously we have described extremes. They do exist, but the majority of us are mixtures, physically and characterologically, of the basic somatotypic elements, with one element prevailing. According to W. H. Sheldon's work, there exist many remarkable relations between body type and, for instance, stomach and duodenal ulcers, type and location of cancers, and heart diseases. E. Kretschmer's findings concerning somatotype and mental illness have been fully confirmed by W. H. Sheldon. Thus, some find that about 60 per cent of schizophrenics are predominantly ectomorphic, whereas manic-depressive patients are overwhelmingly endomorphics. Differences in temperament and character related to somatotype often remain discernible in even the most psychotic patients. The psychiatrist's interest in somatotypes is not only academic, for while it has been shown that hereditary predisposition to schizophrenia does not influence the efficacy of treatment or the outcome of this illness, somatotype does. A young schizophrenic of endomorphic body type tends to have a better prognosis than his ectomorphic fellow-schizophrenic, and the fate of a leptosomatic manic-depressive may well be gloomier than that of a pyknic patient. Naturally one must realize that what has just been described, although substantiated by experiment and clinic, can never be relied on blindly or expected to be correct in all cases. Somatotype is simply one more factor to be reckoned with when we evaluate diagnosis, etiology, and treatment of mental illness.

Physiological Problems:

It is quite easy and probably quite appropriate to make ivory tower statements about mind and body being but one unit. We have become used to hearing that one is unthinkable without the other, that "normal behavior, or for that matter any behavior, depends on normal functioning of the cell unit or neuron in the brain," and that "there is no twisted thought without a twisted molecule." To prove this is another matter.

All over the world, men devoted to research in physiology, electrophysiology, biochemistry, neurophysiology, and related fields, are out to demonstrate this concept. Mountains of data have been accumulated, some of which were hardly printed before they were disproved. Others, apparently irrefutable, are as yet inapplicable. Little by little, an incredibly complex puzzle is being filled in. Serious men in the field believe that in fifty years "the psychiatrist will be the biologically thoroughly sophisticated representative of a mature experimental science."

At this point data are so numerous and contradictory that it would serve no purpose to acquaint the reader with them. Understandably, a great portion of this research is devoted to schizophrenia—still the most frequent practical and theoretical psychiatric problem of our time.

The level at which these research activities are being conducted is mostly the cellular one, i.e., research concerned with individual nerve cells, or neurons, or aggregates of neurons within the brain. A neuron, like any other cell of the body, has a cell membrane which encloses the protoplasm, or cell substance, and the nucleus. In addition, the neuron has extensions of its cell body, fine filaments which carry impulses or messages to and from the cell (dendrites and axons, respectively).

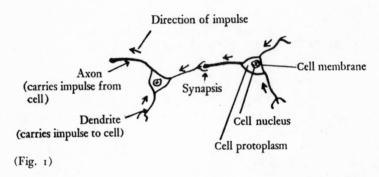

(Fig. 1)

The brain contains many types of neurons, differing in shape, size, and function. Research is concerned with the metabolism of individual neurons. Scientists study the chemical and electrical processes taking place at the cell membrane, which has the capability to determine what shall and shall not enter the cell body. Although these cells are microscopically small, they have been successfully "tapped" with micropipettes, and recordings have been made of their electrical potentials. Through such pipettes, minute amounts of chemical substances, including drugs, have been carried to the immediate vicinity and even inside the cells, and the responses have been recorded. The cell nucleus is also the bearer of the chromosomes we discussed above, which seem to regulate every phase of a person's body metabolism throughout his lifetime. This sheds an entirely new light on the significance of heredity.

Another point of interest is the synapsis, the place where one neuron transmits its impulses to the next. Intricate regulative processes take place at this level. With regard to the functioning of the brain in general and the cell unit in particular, it has become quite obvious that previously cherished ideas and concepts have to be abandoned. Specific regions of the brain have been shown to possess far-reaching regulative functions over metabolism, sleep, mood, feelings, and actions. In animals and men electrical stimulation in these areas, by way of implanted electrodes, produce such conditions as sleep, arousal, mood changes, rage, sexual impulses, and hallucinations. Electrical, biochemical, and hormonal reactions are all intimately involved in these neuronal operations. From experiments it is well known that artificial disturbances of this metabolism can have far-reaching effects on mental activities. Although excessive drinking of alcohol can hardly be called an experiment, it shows clearly the influence on neurons of a toxic substance. The ingestion of minute quantities of a chemical substance called lysergic acid diethylamide, or LSD 25, brings about temporary but profound pathological changes in mental processes resembling those of schizophrenia. In monkeys, the artificial ligation of the large bowel leads to a stuporous condition not unlike the one seen in catatonic schizophrenics. This is thought to be due to self-intoxication with metabolic products that normally would be eliminated. Indeed, it is an interesting fact that most of the toxic substances producing abnormal mental conditions are chemically related to one another and to substances that are normally part of man's metabolism. It is hardly farfetched to hypothesize that minute mistakes in the metabolism of substances regularly produced by the adrenal, thyroid and other glands can lead to toxic products that cause mental derangement.

As mentioned earlier, the handling of "information" within the brain itself is of crucial importance in normal and abnormal behavior, and memory is receiving much attention from the men of the laboratory. It is conceivable that malfunction in this area could explain much of what happens in mental disorders. One theory postulates two kinds of memory: The immediate or fresh memory is constituted by reverberating electrical circuits within a chain of rather few interconnected neurons. These circuits can be tapped at any point and moment. However, within hours after the initial sensory imprint has led to the reverberating circuit, the memory impression is made permanent by the formation of specific molecular albumin structures, constituting the permanent memory. Such a system could explain a variety of phenomena, such as the complete loss of memory for everything immediately preceding a severe blow to the head with unconsciousness. In this instance, the reverberating circuit would be destroyed, and the effect would be the same as when information is lost by a computer being banged on with the fist. The memory is lost because no permanent imprint was made before its destruction. Very old people often remember the names of their schoolteachers but cannot retain new impressions. This could be the consequence of alterations, due to age, in these memory formations. These are some of the thoughts and avenues along which research is conducted in the hope of unlocking the mysteries of mental disorders.

In the preceding paragraphs, we discussed those elements contributing to mental illness which are part of man's biological endowment: heredity and somatotype. We also mentioned physiological or metabolic processes which are partly endowment and partly reaction to external stimuli and stresses such as climate, food, infections, and toxic substances. The latter two in particular are apt to produce mental illness.

Psychological and Environmental Factors:

We now turn our attention to those factors, psychological and sociological in nature, that constitute man's environment, his milieu or the world in which he has to develop, display, and prove himself. They mold man as much as he molds them. They act upon his mental development but implicitly they can also have profound influences on his biological processes. They always remain personal, difficult to evaluate, changing in their emphasis and significance from subject to subject and from observer to observer. What is important to one man may seem insignificant to his neighbor. The physician, endeavoring to understand and treat the sick, must remember that the things he may cherish as desirable, healthy, and good or regard as strange and abnormal may not be so regarded by the patient and his clan.

Man's environment, his private world, consists of the customs and morals of the time, the standard of living and social possibilities, and, more intimately, his mother, father, siblings, spouse, and children. Throughout his life, he never ceases to interact or, as some prefer to say, communicate with his environment. The result of these communications has been called an individual's dynamic development, or his "dynamics." We hesitate to use this word for fear that by now it is half dead of exhaustion from use and abuse. It should convey a feeling of flux, meaningful growth and responses to needs and stresses. It remains somewhat difficult to imagine that earlier men of medicine who used words like character and personality imagined these concepts to be constant, rigid, and static.

Anthropologists, sociologists, behavioral scientists, psychologists, social workers, and psychiatrists are all interested in man's environment and his communications or dealings with it. Large-scale field studies have been conducted here and abroad. Mental illness has been investigated in entire cities and on isolated islands. Our knowledge has been increased and with it the number of unanswered questions. The presumed impact of the environment on the genesis of mental disorders has led some to the exclusive formulation that mental illness is faulty communication. If this definition were to include all the biological, psychological, and environmental factors we have discussed, it would be so broad as to be meaningless. If it intends to emphasize exclusively or primarily the importance of environmental factors at the expense of biological ones its value is dubious.

A concept that has lately received particular attention is that of stress. Stress to an individual can be many things and situations. For instance, the absence of a mother during childhood, or a drinking father; later financial hardship, disappointed love, war or natural catastrophes.

To meet acute stress, an animal either fights or flees, both actions being regulated by and correlated with specific physiological reactions. Man's behavior under comparable conditions does not differ basically from the animals, although for each alternative he has many subtle variations proper to him alone. For man in a crisis, the severity of stress and his strength to overcome it determine whether his fate will be health or mental illness. By strength is meant the sum total of his biological and psychological endowment and his present state of physical and mental health.

Stress as understood here can lead to emotional conflicts and trigger off mental diseases. But it is equally true that it is the necessary ingredient for the development of a normal personality. Only the painful confrontation with reality and limitations, and the constant frictions with his fellow-man, that is, meeting and overcoming stress, can mold an individual capable of holding his own in our world. What may strengthen one may weaken the next, and it may well be that mental illness results only if and when stress and the individual correspond to one another as do key and lock. For instance, one would expect that such prototypes of stress as war and natural disasters would increase the number of the mentally ill, yet this is not the case. Wars have no significant influence on the incidence of schizophrenia and manic-depressive disease, and neuroses and suicides are less frequently encountered during such periods of stress. It is quite true that in many instances our mentally ill come from emotionally and socially unstable families in which, unquestionably, there is much stress. But it is not a rule, and there are no statistics as to the frequency of similar family situations among normal people. Many a famous man and millions of average people have grown up under miserable circumstances. Altogether, it remains amazing how much stress man can actually endure without breaking down, physically or mentally.

A study in a large American city has shown that of all schizophrenic patients admitted to hospitals, more come from slum areas than from the richer residential ones. Does this indicate that schizophrenia is due to poverty, rejection, misery, and other stresses involved in such situations? This remains to be seen. It would be equally simple and possibly equally correct or incorrect to say that those who populate slum areas have drifted into them because mental illness or deficient mental or physical endowment frustrated their efforts to maintain themselves in a better environment. Therefore, one could argue, it is a hereditary and biologically selective process which separates city slums from suburbia. To disentangle such problems might prove to be practically impossible.

Understanding and Explaining:

It appears that man's quest for understanding and explaining is insatiable, and in this respect attempts to teach restraint are discouraging. Yet in psychiatry as elsewhere in science it is important to have a theoretical concept as to what can and what cannot be understood and explained, since understanding is one thing and explaining is another. Explaining implies that a specific cause has a specific effect invariably and logically. For instance, if one hundred normal persons are given intravenous injections of thirty grains of the drug sodium amytal, all will be asleep after a few minutes. There is little room for disagreement. Obviously, the drug causes and therefore explains the sleep. However, if a woman loses her husband and thereupon becomes depressed, we may understand the latter as a reaction to the first, but have we explained it? Is there conclusive, unavoidable evidence of a cause and effect sequence between loss and depression? If we were to find one hundred women who had lost their husbands, it would be rather unlikely to find them all depressed! There is much room for disagreement. Here we are dealing with highly charged motives, most of them embedded in that unknown quantity, the unconscious. As to what has happened within the brains of the ladies who became depressed and those who did not, we can at best make some common sense guesses. We try to understand on the basis of what we are told and of what we remember from similar cases. But beyond this, nothing of certainty can be said.

Let us apply this concept to another psychiatric problem, controversial and heavy with misunderstandings. If a chronic alcoholic drinks to the point of being delirious, he becomes hallucinated, i.e., he may hear the warning or cursing voice of his mother, dead for twenty years, saying that he is doing it again, that he ought to be ashamed of himself. The man's life history may facilitate our understanding of why he hears his mother calling and not his neighbor, but it does not explain the fact that he hallucinates. The alcoholic intoxication of his brain cells, however, does explain their dysfunction and thus the hallucination. This process can be predicted and repeated. Thus, we understand the content of hallucinations from the history, but we explain their appearance biologically. Similarly, we may understand the content of the hallucinations of a schizophrenic patient, but unfortunately we are not able to explain the hallucinations. Sometimes enthusiasm and empathy carry us away. Because we know so well our patient's history and the terrible stresses he has had to go through, we feel certain we have grasped the root of his illness. Soon, however, reality exerts its sobering effect on us. Or does it not?

Another problem in this area is the difficulty of distinguishing between primary and secondary symptoms. We call primary those symptoms unquestionably due to the illness itself, secondary those that are the patient's reactions to his illness. To illustrate: A person had a severe head injury with subsequent epileptic seizures. With each fit he becomes more seclusive and restricted in his activities for fear of having another attack in a public place. The seizure is a primary symptom due to the scar tissue formation in the injured brain. The fear is the patient's reaction to his illness, hence, a secondary symptom. Schizophrenics have primary symptoms, such as thought disorder, emotional ambivalence, and difficulties in relating to others. Long hospitalization will make them dull, apathetic, and lax in their personal hygiene. These symptoms may well be secondary ones, due to neglect, the living conditions in the hospital, and the apparent hopelessness of the situation. If it is possible to avoid hospitalization or to keep it short and to have the patient remain active in some capacity, the secondary symptoms may not develop.

Situations Predisposing to Mental Illness:

We would consider it a justifiable statement, then, that there is not a single social or personal situation or conflict which, invariably, as such, and by itself, would cause or even trigger an emotional disorder. Proceeding from this base line, the question arises as to whether or not there are years, situations or conflicts in a person's life which would fulfill the criteria of our key-and-lock model more than others. Are there years or situations during which a person would be particularly susceptible and sensitive to emotional injuries? Such years and situations, we think, do exist, and in the following chapters the reader will become acquainted with them and their relationships to specific disorders. At this point, only brief mention will be made of a few of them.

The initial information we feed into a computer at the beginning of a program is a decisive factor for its later functioning. Once set, certain patterns are difficult to erase or change without disturbing the entire program. Accordingly, we would expect and find it to be true that a child is most sensitive to his environment during the very first years of his life, when fundamental experiences are being acquired, rules and reaction patterns established, and the foundations of a character being laid. Thus the emotional climate of the home, the predominance of warmth, security and regularity or of impersonal, unpredictable, and hostile behavior of those around him will make permanent imprints in the child. Unlike the computer, the child has to carry on and make the best of a program that has been started with improper information.

René Spitz, an Austrian psychiatrist, has shown clearly what can happen to newborn children of imprisoned mothers if they are brought up in emotionally indifferent nursing homes without a proper substitute for motherly love and care. They may stop eating, show all the signs of a deep depression, and die.

Puberty is another period of heightened sensitivity. Emotional ambivalence, the awakening of sexual desires, and the confrontation with social taboos may lead to erratic behavior and emotional vulnerability. Schizophrenic psychoses appearing at this age often have a particularly poor prognosis.

To women and possibly to men, the menopause is a time of biological and emotional reorientation. At this juncture of life, some encounter difficulties and cannot adjust themselves to the necessary changes. If mental disorders result, they often take the form of paranoid and depressive psychoses, accessible to treatment.

Also, we should mention the beginning senium with the first symptoms of brain atrophy. Forgetfulness and increased fatigability may render the elderly irritable and depressed, if they realize that they can no longer function as they did before. This is very definitely a problem of primary and secondary symptoms. We may not be able to do anything about the former, but much can be done about the latter.

There are other circumstances not to be overlooked, such as prolonged physical illness (tuberculosis), continuous tension and stress (manager's disease), sudden very personal losses and overwhelming experiences (acute adjustment reactions, for instance, during combat), and extreme isolation. The latter can occur on a lonely and boring military mission in the arctic or, experimentally, in "isolation tanks." In these a volunteer is suspended in water and complete darkness. All sensory input is eliminated. Few can tolerate such a situation for more than a few hours. Thinking quickly becomes fragmented and hallucinations may appear. Studies in this area are still in their infant stages but they are promising from a scientific point of view. Such situations may weaken a person's normal regulative defenses against stimuli or stresses from the outside and thus open the path for the appearance of psychic malfunctions.

Common to most of these situations is the occurrence of specific biological changes rendering the individual vulnerable to external stress. How this stress is met depends on the basic personality structure and the prevailing circumstances. For the oversensitive spinster the menopause may pose a grave problem, setting an end to many hopes precariously entertained. For the accomplished mother and wife, the same event may pass unnoticed. Altogether, one does well to remember not so much the small number of those who stumble over these hurdles, but rather the overwhelming number of those who do not.

In closing these remarks on etiology, we hope that some of the basic problems and questions have become visible. We are well-acquainted with the biological, toxic, or infectious causes of some mental disorders, but our present knowledge does not permit the formulation of scientifically satisfactory theories about the genesis of the two major mental illnesses: schizophrenia and manic-depressive disease. Further, it is more than likely that in all mental disorders a host of biological and psychological factors form a closely knit fabric, the overall quality of which decides mental health or illness. Finally, intensive research and experience in this field clearly indicate that there is no room for either complacency or dogmatism.

The Importance of a Diagnosis:

In medicine, in a word or two, a diagnosis symbolizes all that is characteristic of a specific pathological condition. It is a label, and together all medical diagnoses constitute a frame of reference, a framework guaranteeing a certain order in a field that otherwise would be a jungle of vague observations, opinions, and rules.

A diagnosis is based on the presence, not the absence, of symptoms. For instance, it would be improper to conclude that Benjamin, somehow sick and unhappy, must be neurotic because he does not show symptoms of schizophrenia, manic-depressive disease, or brain damage. The concept of neurosis, like any other disease concept, is based on specific criteria, manifested by specific symptoms; if in a given case these are not demonstrable, the diagnosis cannot be made.

There are two sets of reasons why the psychiatrist must make the same effort to establish a diagnosis as does any other physician, or for that matter any person dealing with scientific problems. The first set concerns scientific reasons, the second has to do with the treatment and prognosis of mental illness. To us the two categories are inseparable.

The reader may rightly wonder whether or not this needs to be said. It does. Voices have been raised, particularly in the United States, minimizing and even condemning the search for and the use of diagnoses. It has been claimed that a diagnosis is something sterile and static and that all that matters is prompt and swift treatment of the patient. This viewpoint would be somewhat more comprehensible if all treatments for all psychiatric patients were one and the same—for instance, psychotherapy. But this is not the case. The diagnostic frame of reference presently in use has also been criticized as being impractical, inaccurate, and in many instances unscientific. Any serious psychiatrist will agree with such criticism. But the microscope was not discarded in its infancy because it did not show everything scientists wanted to see. It was refined until it did. To altogether reject a diagnostic order would be unscientific and detrimental to the welfare of the patients.

For the scientist (and a physician is a scientist) it is basic to have a working hypothesis and a frame of reference of well-defined criteria and measures pertaining to his discipline. Both are subject to continuous changes and adaptations according to new factual information emerging from research and experience. Without a frame of reference, scientists of different countries could neither understand each other nor evaluate the results of their own work. The result would be an exercise in futility and duplication.

The psychiatrist who sees only his own schizophrenic patient may well believe him to be unique, incomparable, and not fitting into any diagnostic pigeonhole. Therapeutic luck with some patients and disappointment in others may dispose him to formulate his own therapeutic and prognostic criteria. It can also happen that his concepts of schizophrenia, manic-depressive disease, or neurosis are not shared by many of his colleagues. But a worldwide survey of mental disorders quickly shows that everybody is dealing with about the same problems, that generally applicable rules and criteria can be established, and that information thus gained advances and widens the horizon of our knowledge. Large-scale comparisons of symptomatology, etiology, and particularly therapies and their results are much needed in psychiatry. Obviously, international statistics remain useless unless all concerned apply the same standards, terms, and definitions. Speaking the same scientific language does not, however, imply either proceeding along uniform working hypotheses or using uniform techniques.

This takes us to the second set of reasons. A diagnosis as accurate as possible is a necessity in our daily work. Temporarily, an obsessional neurosis, a beginning schizophrenia, and the initial stage of a tumor in the frontal region of the brain may show very similar symptomatology. If Benjamin has a neurosis, a brain operation would be nonsense and drug therapy useless. He needs psychotherapy. Should he be schizophrenic, psychotherapy might further confuse him, but psychoeffective drugs might re-establish his equilibrium. At this stage, a brain operation would be irresponsible. But should Benjamin have a brain tumor, any treatment short of an operation would be irresponsible. Without treatment, the prognosis for Benjamin the neurotic can be good; for the schizophrenic it is dubious, and for Benjamin with a tumor it is bad. Such problems are common.

Obviously then what the physician needs first of all is a diagnosis. This will permit him to formulate certain expectations and, together with other factors, will direct his thoughts in establishing a treatment plan. Crystallizing a diagnosis out of a host of signs and symptoms is an ancient and noble art; it is not a theoretical nicety, but a grim necessity.

At the beginning of this chapter reference was made to our method of grouping mental disorders. With the exception of certain variations in terminology, there are no basic differences between this scheme and those presently used in civilian and military hospitals in the United States. For didactic reasons we will in the following chapters describe the various diseases in an order that logically proceeds along a theoretical line believed by the author to best represent our present state of knowledge (Fig. 2).

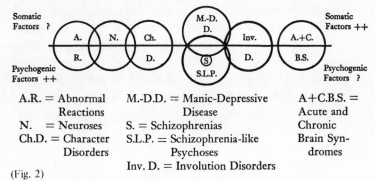

A.R. = Abnormal
       Reactions
N.   = Neuroses
Ch.D. = Character
        Disorders

M.-D.D. = Manic-Depressive
          Disease
S. = Schizophrenias
S.L.P. = Schizophrenia-like
         Psychoses
Inv. D. = Involution Disorders

A+C.B.S. =
Acute and
Chronic
Brain Syn-
dromes

(Fig. 2)

At left we see disorders caused by a maximum of demonstrable psychogenic and a minimum of demonstrable somatic factors. At right will be found diseases caused by a maximum of demonstrable somatic factors and a minimum of psychogenic factors.

Halfway between we place the schizophrenias and manic-depressive disorders. Nothing definite can be said about etiology for either.

The individual disorders or groups of disorders are represented by circles. As can be seen there is some overlapping. Thus, there are transitional cases in which it would be arbitrary to make categorical statements as to the larger diagnostic entity to which they belong. Persons who show transient abnormal emotional reactions to acute and serious stress situations are sometimes basically neurotic or otherwise peculiar. Individuals with character disorders frequently show neurotic symptoms too.

From a diagnostic point of view, the group of schizophrenias is presently the center of much attention and research. There seems to be a well-founded tendency to distinguish between true schizophrenia (inner circle) and schizophrenia-like psychoses (outer circle). The not infrequent overlapping with manic-depressive psychoses may possibly involve only the outer circle. The same may be true for certain cases of involutional depressions and paranoid psychoses. The last circle to the right comprises all disorders that in one way or another are clearly the result of infections, toxic, traumatic, or degenerative processes involving the brain, whether temporary or permanent. It includes most cases of severe mental deficiency.

Summary:

In this chapter an attempt has been made to acquaint the reader with some of the theoretical principles and concepts, thoughts and doubts that pertain to psychiatry as a discipline embracing medical as well as psychological problems. The author realizes that philosophical problems, too, surround this discipline, and are held in high regard by some. We have deliberately restricted our survey to matters as factual and constant as possible, since "psychopathology is concerned with every psychic reality which we can render intelligible by a concept of constant significance" and since "what is needed is a communicable concept for laws and principles."*

We started with definitions of our subject, finding that at present these must remain pragmatic. We divided mental disorders into three groups: disorders that are abnormal variations of normal human experiencing and behavior; diseases caused by known somatic processes; and disorders the etiology of which we know nothing definite about. The model of a modern computer served to demonstrate that where functions along the input-output system can be impaired, psychopathology can arise. This was found to be the case in those processes connecting input with output, concerning reception, interpretation, utilization and storage of information, and last but not least, drive, affect and intellect, as important as they are difficult to understand.

The major part of the chapter was devoted to remarks on etiology, known and suspected and divided into

*Karl Jaspers, *General Psychopathology*. Chicago, University of Chicago Press, 1963.

somatic, biological and environmental, or psychological factors. We tried to show that almost invariably these elements form an intricate unit and that "we have to be content with partial knowledge of an infinity which we cannot exhaust."* Finally we spoke of the need, theoretical and practical, for the formulation of a diagnosis, and proposed a model for dividing mental disorders into groups, an arrangement which we will follow in the subsequent chapters.

To find the way in the maze of certainties and uncertainties that make up today's psychiatry, to follow the path of greatest probability, to arrive at a diagnosis, to draw up a treatment plan and to treat and succeed requires knowledge of what is and can be known, art, and sober intuition. Interpretation cannot be excluded but must be used with restraint. "Science and art of psychiatry always go together—but wherever science has the answer it is preferable to art and intuition."*

*Karl Jaspers, *General Psychopathology*. Chicago, University of Chicago Press, 1963.

·III·

Abnormal Variations of Behavior

(TRANSIENT MALADJUSTMENT REACTIONS, NEUROSES AND CHARACTER DISORDERS)

Introduction:

In this first chapter on individual mental disorders we will discuss disturbances previously introduced as abnormal variations of behavior. We said that the symptoms or behavioral patterns characteristic of these disorders differed quantitatively but not qualitatively from the behavioral patterns of normal persons. Thus, we expect to find exaggerations, diminutions, or caricatures of normal emotions and conduct, but not loss of orientation in time and place, delusions, or hallucinations. The latter symptoms indicate a break with reality. They are of a different quality, and are not found under normal circumstances. We will see them in the functional psychoses and in organic brain diseases.

It must be understood that such a division is theoretical and perhaps somewhat arbitrary. Further research and experience may show a need for correction. Nevertheless, the author believes this distinction to be generally valid and useful.

The disorders under discussion are found on the left side of our scale (Fig. 2). This indicates that in their etiologies environmental and psychological factors seem to predominate, whereas biological ones are difficult to demonstrate or ambiguous. However, as we move from left to right, that is, from the transient maladjustment reactions to the character disorders, genetic predisposition and possibly other somatic disturbances seem to become more influential. There are also marked differences in the responses to treatment. The maladjustment reactions seem to disappear spontaneously after a period of rest with some verbal encouragement. Many neuroses abate spontaneously or respond well to psychotherapy, a few remain therapy-resistant. Most character disorders, however, are unresponsive to the treatment methods presently available.

Transient Maladjustment Reactions:

Definition: Under this term are grouped sudden, short-lasting pathological but nonpsychotic behavioral changes in otherwise normal persons under excessive stress.

Commentary: The word "sudden" indicates that these conditions usually develop within hours or days, particularly in connection with gross stress, such as catastrophes. Also included, however, are reactions to more insidious situations, such as unexpected changes in a family constellation, difficult transitions in the style of life, the arrival of a step-parent, the beginning of puberty, or retirement. In these instances, symptomatology may develop more gradually. By "short-lasting" we understand that the disorders will abate within days or weeks, i.e., after the shock of a catastrophe has been overcome, or more gradually within months when an adjustment has been made to a new situation. If the condition persists it is likely that other pathogenic factors are at play and that a different diagnosis is indicated.

"Pathological, but nonpsychotic behavioral changes" are alterations in a person's behavior that are unexpected, inappropriate, and ineffectual in solving the crisis at hand. Often they are unconventional or socially unacceptable, but the symptoms, such as flight, tantrums, nail-biting, or apathy and inefficiency, do not reach psychotic proportions. The patient does not lose contact with reality, does not develop symptoms characteristic of psychoses as we have mentioned above.

"Excessive stress" is a relative and subjective concept that cannot be defined uniformly. A roller coaster means fun to some and extreme anxiety to others. The dull noise of approaching bombers may either paralyze or alert. In a marriage, a single word can open an abyss carefully covered for decades. We have discussed this problem before and will encounter it time and again. It is an important issue. At best we can say that an excessive stress is a stress which, for one reason or another, an individual cannot tolerate.

Physically and mentally healthy people usually adjust themselves in some acceptable form to the ordinary adversities of life. Indeed, it is often astounding how fast and completely they adjust to situations previously or afterwards thought to be intolerable and inhuman. In moments of danger and distress, some laugh and others cry, some fight, some recede and others comply. There are people so emotionally stable, so secure and sure of themselves, that neither earthquake nor months of intense fighting in jungles will disturb their equanimity. Others, less fortunate, have to make great efforts to adapt themselves to new and unexpected situations.

But natural catastrophes, like tornadoes, inundations, earthquakes, or conditions in modern war, man's self-imposed hell on earth, and other dramatic situations, may at times disrupt the well-established defense patterns of people who were not expected to lose their composure. Or were they? This question, we believe, is debatable, and again we prefer to think in terms of our lock-and-key model. During his entire life a person may adjust well to difficulties of all kinds, except for the one time that he encounters a situation that somehow touches on repressed emotional conflicts he cannot master, once they are strongly evoked. What we suggest is that many of those who react to stress with transient disruptions of their normal behavioral patterns have some basic emotional weakness which, under ordinary circumstances, never manifests itself. For all practical purposes these persons are not mentally ill.

Clinical Manifestations:

Transient situational maladjustment reactions occur at all ages. They are particularly frequent during the earlier years of life. Normal behavior in infants and children depends very much on a well-regulated life style with as few rules as possible. It is only in the process of growing up that man becomes flexible by developing a variety of behavioral patterns which allow him to adjust himself to the frequently changing demands of his environment. In unexpected, unfavorable, emotionally traumatic situations, children often react with misbehavior quickly and in a seemingly exaggerated fashion. With equal suddenness they may revert back to normal conduct, once the difficulties have been overcome.

To journeys, temporary absence of the mother, irregular feeding patterns or other upsetting circumstances, normal babies may react with excitability or apathy, with refusal to eat, drink, and sleep. During childhood, symptoms such as nail-biting, thumb-sucking, bed-wetting, and masturbation may be the responses to lack of consistency, neglect, or exaggerated demands on the part of the parent or to other events which create anxiety and insecurity in the child. As the child grows older, his acting out becomes more colorful and, to the parents and community, more alarming. Truancy may be the expression of fear of a teacher, a threatening classmate or a difficult academic subject. It may also be the child's way of hitting back at a parent. Stealing is frequently a sign of emotional deprivation and the same may be true for destructiveness, cruelty, and sexual offenses. There are no rules that indicate the cause of any given type of acting out. Only careful study of the individual case can provide the answer.

In adolescence, new roots for difficulties appear. With the maturing of sexual drives, emotional turmoil and ambivalence arise toward members of the same or the opposite sex. Impulses and desires clash with parental, religious, and other taboos. Moodiness and erratic behavior, suicidal gestures and symptoms ensue, resembling those found in neuroses and character disorders. These reactions are often dramatic, puzzling, and frightening. Yet, as quickly as they appear, they also vanish. To the relief or disappointment of those around him, the adolescent rebel or the promising artist settles down to the pedestrian life of the average citizen.

The classic type of a transient maladjustment reaction in adult life is the acute emotional faltering of the soldier on the battlefield. Many of such cases have been observed during the last two world wars and the Korean action. The sudden crises were characterized by uncontrollable trembling and shaking, or weakness and paralysis in the extremities, by sobbing and crying, and panic reactions such as crawling out of the trench or standing up in an unprotected area.

As to the treatment of these casualties, an important lesson was learned during the second world war. Quick removal of the soldier from the immediate battle scene and a short period of rest right behind the lines proved to be highly successful. After a night or two in a bed, a shower, a shave, a warm meal, and a good talk with the psychiatrist, the minister, or any other understanding person, most of these soldiers regained their composure and returned to their units. Removal to more distant hospitals with prolonged stay, as practiced earlier, often led to chronic emotional casualties. Shame and guilt feelings over the abandoning of buddies at the moment of greatest danger were some of the principal reasons for the unfortunate development in these cases.

Finally, there are the adjustment reactions in late life. Similar to those in childhood and adolescence, they are the results of a poorly mastered encounter between physiological changes (menopause, beginning senium) and demands for new adaptations in a changing environment. It sometimes needs a wise heart to endure the emptiness of a house that used to be filled with the business and laughter of children. The deaths of loved ones come more frequently, reminding the elderly of who might be next. Also, idleness after a busy life is not as easily tolerated as many think while they are still working. The serenity of the old may be preceded by a period of grouchiness, depression, and irritability, and by the accentuation and caricature of the more unpleasant traits of a personality.

The Neuroses:

Definition: A neurosis is an emotional disorder belonging to the category of abnormal variations of behavior. Usually the symptoms are circumscribed, leaving personality and intellectual functions intact. The cause is an emotional conflict, the nature of which remains unconscious. In most cases, the neurotic person realizes that he is sick. The course of the untreated neurosis is a chronic one, but spontaneous remissions occur. Theoretically, the treatment of choice is psychotherapy.

Commentary: The meaning of the first sentence of this definition has been clarified.

"Symptoms are circumscribed." It will be seen that in character disorders the entire personality is involved in the morbid development, as reflected in a diffuse and general inability to function under certain circumstances. In manic-depressive disease, schizophrenia, and the involutional psychoses, the fully developed illness does not affect intellectual functions as such, but often prevents their proper use. What these patients exhibit is a travesty of their normal personality and mode of functioning. This is also true in patients with serious brain damage, where intellectual faculties are impaired as well.

In neuroses or, as they are also called, in psychoneuroses, specific functions or behavior are affected, often only under certain circumstances. For instance, in a social gathering, in a shop or on a street, a neurotic person may not show any unusual behavior, whereas each morning he spends two hours trying to decide which pair of socks to wear. Everyday a most efficient business executive may climb the five flights of stairs to his office because he is afraid of elevators. These are two of a great number of phobias, compulsions, obsessions, and other isolated symptoms to be discussed below.

However, there are persons with an all-pervasive neurotic anxiety which paralyzes their functioning in society; and an isolated phobia can also become a crippling disorder. A person with an insurmountable fear of germs may finally stop leaving his room for fear of catching a fatal disease. In a conversation these neurotics often prove to be charming, intelligent, rational, and relevant. In some, however, the exclusive preoccupation with their fears and rituals may lead to a secondary obliteration of the personality.

"The cause is an emotional conflict." The neurosis has been called the only true or primary disease of the mind, because it is the only emotional disorder which is clearly, and for some exclusively, defined as a reaction of the psyche to an unbearable emotional conflict. Here, understanding and explaining would be synonymous, i.e., the dynamic conflict, which we understand, would be the sole causative agent, thus explaining the existence of the neurosis. Again, the author prefers to think in terms of the lock-and-key model and joins those who hold that even for the genesis of a neurosis a constitutional liability or predisposition is necessary.

This predisposition has been described as a general genetic lack of vitality, or asthenia, or as a primary emotional vulnerability. Other authors have spoken of an insufficiency in the highest regulative cerebral functions, whereby lower, more primitive functions would be released or disinhibited. Such concepts remain vague and await physiological verification. Nevertheless it is true that emotionally abnormal personalities are more frequently found in the families of neurotics than in the average population.

As to the emotional trauma or the neurotic conflict, it was thought originally that a single emotionally traumatic event, experienced in childhood, triggers the neurotic development. For instance, the child who happened to observe his parents during the act of intercourse could be overwhelmed and frightened by the experience. He would become sensitized to sexual provocations and would react to them with fear and flight for years to come.

Presently it is more commonly accepted that a series of similar traumatic events will cause the neurotic sensitization and development. It is also held that the event does not have to be of a sexual nature and that the sensitization does not have to occur in childhood only, as was formerly believed.

It is more significant that the traumatic events are unexpected, unwelcome, and apt to trigger emotional feelings, desires or reactions that are unacceptable in a given situation. For these reasons, they invariably arouse anxiety. For example, the son, preoccupied in a diffuse way with sexual problems and particularly attached to the mother, may experience tumultuous emotions at the unexpected sight of the parents' intercourse. Fear of the mother being attacked, an impulse to help her, and, simultaneously, jealousy toward the father and the desire to be in his place may be aroused. Particularly the last two emotions would be disturbing and unacceptable. Further events of a similar nature might deepen the emotional confusion. In another instance, a woman during menopause, prudish but thought to be happily married, may fall in love with an employer who represents all those male traits she always had professed to despise. The result may be a medley of sexual desires, shame, and disgust, of love and an awareness of social taboos.

In one way or another, the traumatic events would be a shock with which the individual is not prepared to deal on a conscious level. Defense mechanisms have to be mobilized.

There are various ways of dealing with unpleasant events, threatening emotions and conflicts between instincts, drives and moral codes. As mentioned before, in the face of an external threat it is possible to either fight or flee. The same solutions exist as to internal threats. For the lady in love, a mature way of handling herself might be to sit down and think and wonder about her life and the present situation, and to find a rational solution to her dilemma. Or, if she has the courage for adventure, nothing to lose and something to gain, she may shed her former life as a snake does its skin and embark on a new one. Whether or not she will fare better than the snake, whose new skin very much resembles the old one, is another question. In both instances, she manages or fights the problem on a conscious level.

By contrast, the neurotic way of handling emotional turmoil is by fleeing, the basic mechanism of which is forgetting. Everybody has this ability to simply forget something disagreeable, to push it out of his conscious mind down into the unconscious. However, and this is essential, in the neurotic this defense mechanism will not serve its purpose of restoring peace and harmony. Indeed, the forgetting or repressing of an emotional conflict can only be a pseudo-solution. For many people pseudo-solutions are quite acceptable, but a sensitive and insecure individual with strong desires, weak controls, and an alert conscience cannot deceive himself so easily without suffering. In such a person, a restlessness or anxiety arises. The feelings stirred up but repressed seek expression, and since they are not acceptable in their original form they reemerge in disguise. The type of disguise determines the type of neurosis.

"In most cases the neurotic person realizes that he is sick." Unlike most schizophrenic patients, the neurotic person has an acute awareness of being ill. What he fears, what he is compelled to do, he realizes to be foreign to his personality and unreasonable. He suffers and seeks help.

A neurosis often develops over a period of many years, having its roots in childhood, and complicating life to the end. That this is not always true has been demonstrated by some of the few existing statistics regarding the neuroses. For instance, a study in England showed that half the neurotic patients placed on a waiting list for psychotherapy declared that they no longer needed treatment when their names finally came up for therapy. Frequently neurotic reactions that develop later in life disappear spontaneously after weeks, months, or a few years. It is obvious that such spontaneous cures render the evaluation of therapy extremely difficult.

Treatment will be dealt with in the chapter on management. At this point it may suffice to say that since by definition the neurosis is caused by a psychological conflict, the ideal therapy would have to consist of uncovering this conflict.

Clinical Manifestations:

Neurotic reactions have been classified in various ways. Some authors distinguish between character neuroses and situational neuroses. The first originate in childhood and influence the development of the entire personality. The latter crystallize around an acute stressful life situation at a more advanced age, and thus remain more peripheral with respect to the personality. To this group would belong the traumatic neuroses that develop after physical injuries sustained under dramatic circumstances like automobile accidents and war situations. In these cases the motive of gain is particularly prominent if compensation from insurance companies can be expected, and it is often difficult to disentangle unconscious or truly neurotic motivations from shrewd malingering.

Another approach, followed by the United States statistical manual on mental disorders, consists in classifying the neuroses according to their most prominent symptom, for example, neurotic anxiety reactions, obsessive-compulsive, and depressive reactions.

A particular category of disorders which attracts much attention today is that of the psychosomatic illnesses. Indeed, there is much talk about psychosomatic medicine, as if it were a newly discovered and independent branch of medicine. But psychosomatic medicine is as old as the knowledge of medicine; it has always been practiced and it would hardly be original to call the entire field of medicine psychosomatic, since there is practically no illness or therapy that does not involve both body and psyche. In psychiatry we specifically call psychosomatic or psycho-physiologic those disorders in which somatic symptoms are expressions of emotional conflicts as defined in this chapter. For instance, heart palpitations or a stomach ulcer would be seen as the disguises in which repressed anxiety reappears on the surface.

The decision to place an individual case in one or another of the subgroups of neuroses is frequently an arbitrary one. Most neurotic patients show symptoms of various sub-groups. In the context of this book, it would serve no purpose to go into detailed descriptions of all the different neurotic reactions. A general account of some of the outstanding clinical symptoms will be more rewarding.

The least disguised expression of unconscious anxiety is a conscious, but to the patient unexplainable, diffuse anxiety arising at unspecific moments. It may be accompanied by vague expectations of danger and somatic symptoms like tremulousness, diarrhea, or a constant need for food.

In contrast to this, anxiety can be localized in time, place, and situation, that is, it may arise only in specific situations. For instance, our executive may refuse to ride the elevator because each time he does use it he experiences a severe anxiety attack. Such a reaction is called a phobia (Greek: fear). Other phobias may concern germs, crossing a street, or even the pronouncing of certain words.

Together with phobias or by themselves, we frequently encounter obsessions and compulsions. A neurotic may have to go through tedious rituals each time he goes to bed. Another may be compelled to count telephone poles on his way to work, to return several times to his house to reassure himself that he locked the door, or may have to wash his hands so frequently that the skin breaks. Another patient may be obsessed with ideas, thoughts, or obscene words he does not wish to think of.

The only manifestation of a neurosis can be a depression. Unlike the depressive phase of a manic-depressive disorder, which is usually recurrent and difficult to relate to a specific incident, the neurotic depressive reaction follows a definite saddening event, like the death of a family member or friend. To the observer, however, this depression would appear to be out of proportion to the loss, would last longer than normal mourning and the patient's feelings and self-accusations would seem to be unwarranted. Analysis of such cases might show that the patient's feelings toward the lost object were very ambivalent, a mixture of love and hate. It is difficult to admit hate toward a just deceased person whom one was supposed to have loved. This creates vivid guilt feelings and anxiety, and the neurotic reacts to these with denial, forgetting, or repression. The result is a depression which really is an unconscious overcompensation or an answer to the repressed guilt feelings.

Finally, we mention the conversion reactions. They are not seen as often today as a few decades ago. In these cases anxiety manifests itself in the form of pseudo-somatic or functional symptoms, such as paralysis of extremities or inability to speak. Physical examination does not reveal any somatic defect. Motives of secondary gain and symbolic meanings of the symptoms seen in almost all neuroses are particularly obvious in these conversion reactions. By secondary gain we mean that the illness serves a certain purpose for the patient, such as saving him from a disagreeable situation or securing insurance benefits. However, the patient is not conscious of such connections. For instance, a girl who has a date which she both desires and fears may suddenly complain of weakness or paralysis in her legs. She is bedfast. The doctor arrives, shakes his head, and miraculously cures the girl the day after the date has been postponed indefinitely. Secondary gain, as well as the symbolic meaning of the symptom, is obvious.

Addiction to alcohol or drugs can be the neurotic's attempt to relieve anxiety, but more often, addicts have serious character disorders. We will speak about them under that heading.

Theoretical Concepts:

The neurotic reaction is the only mental disorder that includes psychodynamic concepts as an integral part of the definition. It is also the only entity that merits the term "reaction," since it is thought to be the reaction of a person's psyche to an emotional conflict. In the absence of a conflict a diagnosis of neurotic reaction cannot be sustained.

From a theoretical or psychodynamic point of view, and in the broadest possible terms, the neurotic reaction might be called a failure in a person's attempt to master an emotional crisis. The crisis itself is thought to be the result of a clash of desires or instinctual drives within the personality with forces geared toward their inhibition. This inhibition causes anxiety. If the control is unsuccessful, as in neuroses, substitutive symptom-formations are the result.

The literature of psychiatry abounds in theories with regard to the genesis and meaning of neurotic reactions. Most of the modern psychodynamic theories were conceptualized on the basis of knowledge or inferences gained from analysis of neurotic patients; subsequently, they were to include other mental disorders. We have pointed out earlier some of the fallacies inherent in these theories. We will briefly mention the principal concepts involving neuroses. All of them are very much the fruits of philosophical concepts of man's nature and destiny their founders had. According to Freud's psychoanalysis, man is basically an animal driven by instincts. His aim is the avoidance of pain and the search for pleasure, which means the satisfaction of his sexual desires. The sexual instincts, or the libido, constitute the fuel for his life. Art and intellectual and spiritual goals are seen as transformed or sublimized libido, which, due to social restrictions, cannot consume itself to its natural limits. The nucleus of the neurosis lies in the struggle between libido and taboo, disturbed through emotional shock at a specific phase of a child's development.

Psychoanalytical theories have undergone marked but not radical changes. In their claim to provide a comprehensive frame of reference for the understanding of mental development and illness they remain controversial, as do other psychodynamic theories.

Alfred Adler, at first a disciple of Freud, embraced another concept of man. According to him, the mainspring of life is man's need to assert himself in order to overcome actual or fancied insufficiencies in his personality or physical structure. To escape the necessity of proving his power the neurotic makes "arrangements," i.e., he flees into illness, becomes guilty and anxious, and thus neurotic symptoms or excuses ensue.

Lately, existential analysis has received some attention in this country. Existential analysis, based on very specific philosophical concepts, originated in Europe. Its chief proponents, Ludwig Binswanger, Erwin Straus, and Medard Boss, are primarily concerned with man's spiritual aspirations, which they hold to be as basic as his animalistic ones. For them, man's purpose is to develop all his potentials to the point where he can transcend himself, or exist in a perfect, unselfish communion with another human being. Man is not so much driven by instincts: he has a free will, and with this is responsible for himself. Man is seen as the only living being who takes cognizance of his own development and is able to take a position with regard to this development. Indeed, he not only can but must take a position in order to fulfill his human responsibility. The neurotic, dishonest toward himself, falls short in his attempt to take a positive part in his growing up. This failure results in guilt and anxiety and in neurotic symptom-formation,

In a previous chapter we mentioned the reflex and learning theories based on the work of Ivan Pavlov. They apply well to neurosis. From the example of the dog one can see that it is possible to provoke a neurosis experimentally by first creating and then disturbing patterns of behavior. Similar experiments have been made with other laboratory animals. However, one of the crucial questions remains: Is it admissible to apply results from animal experiments to man? The answer of the existentialist is a clear "no."

Obviously, some of these theories are earthy, others lofty. Whether or not any of them contains truth is difficult to decide. But when we speak of man's destiny, what is truth? Indeed, it may be that this word is out of place and what is really meant are values. What is of value, only the individual can determine. Is the neurosis a problem of values or a problem of somatic processes? Can it really be explained or be understood? The answer is not yet available.

A Case:

A woman, married, forty years of age, complains of headaches, back pains, and stomach pain. She is constantly on edge, worried; she sleeps poorly and at night often awakens from terrifying nightmares. Whenever her husband is late from work she suffers agonies, believing that something terrible must have happened to him. At the sight of a policeman she breaks out in cold sweat and her heart pounds. She is sexually unsatisfied. The home situation is secure, the husband understanding, her suffering is respected.

The patient does not have any intellectual deficit, she thinks clearly, she has no delusions or hallucinations. She realizes that her fears and her nervousness are not warranted, but she cannot stop them. Day and night she thinks about her past. This past was tranquil and harmonious until the patient was 16 years of age. At that time she was taken to a German concentration camp, and for the next five years her life was constantly in danger. Her parents were shot in her presence, she was beaten, humiliated, hungry, and clad in rags. Only two thoughts kept her going: How best to hide and how to find an extra piece of bread. She survived, but when the holocaust was over she found that everybody in her family had died, that her house was destroyed. Life would never be as it had been before, as she had hoped it would be. At that point she gradually developed the described symptoms. She felt vaguely that it was not right for her to have survived while everybody else had perished. She felt guilty when she could have been comfortable and her fears of doom grew again. There was a chance for her to get a considerable sum of money for compensation; she desired it but it did not make her happy when she thought of her parents.

This history does not need much commentary. The elements are part of a traumatic neurosis. It is a neurosis typical of concentration camp survivors: a healthy background and then years of severe physical and emotional stress. Symptoms appear when the silent hopes for a revival of the past are shattered and combine with guilt feelings over the individual's own survival. Instead of looking forward the patient remains oriented toward the past which she cannot digest. Symptoms rich in symbolic meaning are predominant, with anxiety the central one. The possible financial compensation may contribute to the persistence of the symptoms.

·IV·

The Character Disorders

(PSYCHOPATHIES)

"Indignation, though on the whole
a useful social force,
becomes harmful when it is directed
against victims of maladies
that only medical skill can cure."

BERTRAND RUSSELL

Introduction:

The character disorders—they are also referred to as psychopathies or psychopathic personalities—constitute the last group of disorders belonging to the abnormal variations of behavior. In this book all three designations shall be used synonymously. The originally neutral term "psychopathy," still used in Europe, has acquired a derogatory connotation in the United States. In our official nomenclature it has been replaced by the term "character disorders."

It is difficult to draw a distinctive line between neuroses and character disorders. There is much overlapping. We often see primarily psychopathic personalities with neurotic symptoms and predominantly neurotic patients with a psychopathic character.

No other psychiatric client has engendered as much passionate controversy as has the psychopath. Living as he does in the borderland between health and illness, he has never ceased to arouse the ire and malevolent attention of those around him. A dispassionate discussion is in order.

Since we are speaking of character disorders it is appropriate to briefly define what is meant by the term "character." There are uncounted numbers of such definitions. Essentially, the author will follow Karl Jaspers who uses the terms personality and character synonymously.

Character is the totality of how a person experiences and expresses himself, how he moves, loves and hates, how he conquers and suffers, what goals and ideals he chooses, what he does with them, and what he does with himself. Implicit in this definition is the individual's awareness of himself as an individual.

Ludwig Klages distinguishes between the formal structure and the qualities of a character. The first comprises: (1) temperament (speed of arousal, strength, and persistence of feelings); (2) the predominant mood or affect, varying between sadness and euphoria; (3) the formal attributes of volition (strength, a weakness of willpower, energy, spontaneity of acting, tenacity, obstinacy). By qualities of a personality Klages meant the system of drives and instincts, or the actual substance or essence of the character.

Character is partially given at birth. It has a geno-typical, biological foundation which cannot be understood in psychological terms but which carries the structure of understandable meaningful psychic connections. Thus, a character reveals itself; equally, it develops and is the result of a development in time. It is formed by what the world brings to the individual or withholds from him. In this sense, the character of a person must be read in his biography. The foundation of the character includes the freedom of possibilities to develop, but this freedom limits research, it cannot be the object of research. Crossing these limits, we leave empiricism and enter the realm of ideal types of personalities, which are a matter for philosophy.

As scientists we observe the manifestations of a character, but beyond all that is meaningful and understandable man cannot be grasped but only encountered as one human existence by another. In man there is always a residue which we cannot understand.

A characterology can be based on ideal personality types, that is, on philosophical constructions hardly ever met in life, or on real types. The latter are modeled after clinical observations and intuition. As has been mentioned earlier, there seem to be close links between somatotype and character. The reader who wishes to learn about personality types will be more rewarded by reading great literature than by studying psychological or philosophical textbooks. Don Quixote, Sancho Panza, Raskolnikov, or Anna Karenina are characters we never cease to recognize in those around us.

What constitutes a normal or an abnormal personality

cannot be a matter of statement but only of evaluation. Personality characteristics vary according to the degree of unity or the amount of scatter in the meaningful elements in a given individual. The more scattered and disconnected these elements are, the more abnormal the individual. The same can be expressed if we speak of the equilibrium and harmony of a personality or of polarities and their synthesis. The more disharmony there is in a character, or the less synthesis, the more abnormality we will encounter.

Definition: Character disorders manifest themselves by excessive but nonpsychotic variations in one or several dimensions of behavior. They are apparent throughout an entire lifespan, and have a tendency to cause society to suffer from them. Their etiology is unknown, most likely multifactorial. Treatment is difficult.

Typology: Psychopathic personalities have been described and classified in many different ways. Normal characters vary unendingly and so do their abnormal variations, and arranging them in a typology is a questionable procedure. But some order is necessary and a certain agreement can be reached on some major groups of personality types oriented around the most prominent clinical symptoms. For instance, we can speak of schizoid, cyclothymic, or paranoid psychopaths, if the individuals present primarily symptoms of hypersensitivity and isolation, of frequent mood swings, or symptoms of a persecutory nature. Further, we would describe the passive and dependent, the aggressive, the asocial and antisocial characters. An arbitrary number of other types and subtypes could be added to these without increasing the accuracy of the system. However, instead of describing such types we will aim at a more basic delineation by returning to the elements of the character structure.

The differences between one type of psychopathic personality and another can be understood as dysfunctions in the specific spheres of the character, such as temperament and mood, willpower and motivation, or feelings, drives, and instincts. Infrequently, however, would we find a psychopath showing dysfunctions in one of these areas only. This is one reason why classifications are rejected by some psychiatrists.

Clinical manifestations of dysfunctions in mood and temperament are abnormal depressive or euphoric dispositions, frequent or inconsistent mood swings, explosivity or shallowness of temperament. Abnormal variations in willpower and motivations produce people who are either extremely weak- or strong-willed, and show very little persistence in their plans and endeavors, or are abnormally tenacious, unreasonable and inflexible in the pursuit of a single cause. Most paranoid psychopaths and fanatics belong to the last category.

The most serious social consequences stem from dysfunction or abnormal dispositions in the areas of basic drives. In this respect, sexual aberrations and a person's inability to sympathize with others, to have empathy or to love deserve special mentioning. The results of such dysfunctions can be seen in the asocial and antisocial delinquents. What is so puzzling and frightening about many of these is the seeming ease with which they proceed from one criminal act to the next, from stealing a bicycle to fraud and murder, without ever showing concern for their victims. This lack of empathy, together with the inability to learn from past experiences, is typical of psychopathic personalities. These qualities often make them immune to therapy and administrative correction.

Abnormal variations in sexual drives in a psychopathic person are often a serious concern to the community. Without embarking on a discussion of the moral merits and issues of such concerns, it is necessary to state that serious sexual perversions, such as homosexuality, exhibitionism, or voyeurism can be expressions of serious character disorders or other mental disorders. If so, they are primarily medical problems and cannot be changed, cured, or suppressed by social verdict or incarceration. However, great caution must be exercised in calling one or the other sexual activity abnormal. Personal and cultural bias and preconceptions are serious obstacles to an objective study and discussion of these problems. The Kinsey Report,* after an exhaustive study of an immense amount of data, concludes as follows: "No type of sexual behavior in human beings can be considered 'abnormal' or 'unnatural' and if it were not for training to the contrary almost every person would indulge in almost every type of sexual behavior." Thus, what is "normal" and "abnormal" becomes a question of individual control and adherence to a socially acceptable pattern.

With regard to homosexuality, it must be remembered that not everybody can be called homosexual who once or twice in his life has had a homosexual experience. Fleeting homosexual feelings and experimental activities are part of

*Alfred C. Kinsey, et al. *Sexual Behavior in the Human Female.* Philadelphia, W. B. Saunders & Co., 1953.

the normal process of growing up. Under unusual circumstances, as in prisons, or in the military service during wartime, homosexual acts are committed by persons who are exclusively heterosexual under normal conditions. Homosexuality has existed throughout the ages and in all cultures of the world. In many ethnic groups it has been and still is accepted as a normal form of sexual behavior. Overt homosexual activities can be observed in many species of animals. With this information in mind, we define the homosexual as a person who is persistently, exclusively, or primarily attracted, emotionally and physically, to members of the same sex. To this we have to add that recent research shows the possible existence of genetic aberrations with consequent significant physiological hormonal variants in body metabolism.

Most homosexuals live a quiet, inconspicuous life, alone or with a companion. Many are married. Great artists and statesmen and successful businessmen have been homosexuals. Merely on account of their sexual abnormality, homosexuals are of neither lower nor higher moral standards than their nonhomosexual contemporaries. If they are more exposed to blackmail and thus become "security risks" this is primarily the consequence of the general negative and vindictive attitude of the public toward homosexuality.

The exhibitionist is a person who inappropriately exposes his genitals to members of the opposite sex. Typical of this is the young man, usually fearful of women, who on a lonely road opens his pants at the sight of some little girls or of a passing woman. The voyeur tries to remain unseen while he looks through windows or keyholes to see a woman undress. There are many other forms of sexual perversions, some benign and practiced only in privacy, others serious, involving seduction of children, rape, and murder. Their common feature is the weakness, excess, or distortion of the pervert's sexual drives, which makes it impossible for him to satisfy his sexual needs in a normal way. Not infrequently, too, abnormal fluctuations in mood are found in these persons, as well as lack of willpower to resist temptation and of empathy for the victims of the abnormal sexual acts.

Another group of psychopathic personalities are the addicts. Whereas the alcohol addict, or alcoholic, seems to enjoy the benign approval of his contemporaries, the drug addict merely incites their scorn and fear. An addict is one who in an attempt to alleviate a disagreeable state of mind cannot resist taking alcohol or certain drugs in quantities and frequencies that will ultimately harm his physical and mental health. The drugs involved are primarily the various barbiturates and opium derivatives and components containing the stimulating amphetamines, such as Dexedrine.

In most addicts the basic dysfunctions are abnormal fluctuations in mood, primarily in the sense of mild subclinical depressions. Consequently, these people often feel lonely, worthless, tired, and diffusely sick, and in trying to escape from their misery they start to drink or to use drugs. Conflicts in the home, themselves often the results of mood disturbances or of other character inadequacies, may trigger off the addiction. At other times it is the sleeping pill, the sedative, or the reducing medicine prescribed by the physician which paves the way for an addiction. Physicians and nurses, having easy access to drugs, constitute a high percentage of the drug addicts. Since the organism adapts itself quickly to drugs, ever-increasing doses of the medication are needed to bring about "peace of mind."

Lack of willpower, defeating the good intentions to stop the habit of taking a drink or a pill, may help in establishing and reinforcing the addiction. Also, when used over a certain length of time addictive drugs and alcohol destroy the fine structure of the nerve cells in the brain. This leads to further alterations of character, as manifested by increasing intellectual and emotional dullness, apathy, irritability, and ethical decline. Thus a vicious circle is established, which, over a period of many years of misery for both the addict and his environment, leads to the unhappy end in idleness and oblivion in a mental hospital of so many of the alcohol and drug addicts.*

Hardly ever can a single factor, somatic or environmental, be considered the sole cause of a character disorder. As mentioned before, a character is partially determined at birth. As a matter of fact, signs of abnormal behavior can be observed during the very first months of life of a child who later develops a distinct character disorder. The predetermination can be seen as a genetic predisposition or as the result of physiological brain injury during gestation or at the time of delivery. It is conceivable that infections or other diseases that the mother has during pregnancy may influence the development of the fetus' brain. Prolonged labor or an umbilical cord strung around the baby's neck can impair the cerebral blood circulation, causing insufficient oxygenation and permanent brain damage.

Infectious diseases involving the brain during the first

---

*The psychotic disorders resulting from chronic alcoholism will be discussed in Chapter VI.

years of life, such as encephalitis, can result in permanent mental disorders presenting all the features of a character disorder. In these cases, we may see disinhibition of sexual impulses, irritability, and emotional instability, together with perfect preservation of all intellectual faculties. If the encephalitis is properly diagnosed, the described symptoms will be considered as belonging to a chronic organic brain syndrome secondary to encephalitis. (See Chapter VI.) In other words, the symptoms are the consequence of irreversible brain damage. It is tempting to assume that many psychopathic personalities have received some brain damage due to mild toxic or infectious diseases that were never diagnosed. The fact that abnormal encephalographic records are being found in a much higher percentage among psychopaths than among the normal population may lend support to this assumption.

Other factors responsible for the shaping of character disorders must be sought for in the environment in which the child grows up. Emotional insecurity, unreliability of the parents, and exposure to physical or emotional mistreatment can help distort the image the child forms of the world around him and condition his responses to it. An already vulnerable brain may well be less resistive to such nefarious influences and less able to correct early responses in the light of later and better experiences.

Various psychodynamic theories try to understand which particular environmental constellations will lead to such specific abnormal reactions as, for instance, homosexuality. Although frequently enlightening, these theories must remain conjectural. In the literature index the reader will find the titles of pertinent articles on this subject. The impressions gained from such dissertations have to be balanced with the knowledge of results from genetic studies. Franz Kallman, for example, reports a 100 per cent concordance for homosexuality in one-egg twins as against 11 per cent in two-egg twins. (Concordance indicates the twins' chances for the demonstration of identical traits.) However, comparative figures found by other researchers are considerably lower. It is difficult to explain this wide gap between the incidence of homosexuality in monozygotic and heterozygotic twins on the basis of environmental influences alone.

In conclusion: A character disorder is the result of the development of a personality. This development cannot be understood solely on the basis of dysfunctions of drives or mood. It is always the sum total of interactions between what is given at birth or any other moment in life, and what is experienced. The result is an attitude toward the world that can be positive, open and constructive, or negative, hostile and destructive.

Laboratory Studies and Statistics:

In all disorders belonging to the abnormal variations of behavior routine laboratory studies (blood tests, urine analysis, liver function tests, electrocardiogram, X-ray studies) at present fail to demonstrate findings characteristic of any particular clinical symptoms or syndromes. The only exception is the electroencephalogram, which is often diffusely abnormal in psychopathic personalities, particularly in those of the criminal types. It may also show patterns indicative of epilepsy in persons who are clinically not epileptics but who exhibit excessive irritability, moodiness, and explosive, often destructive behavior.

With regard to statistics, it has already been mentioned that an assessment of the frequency of the occurrence of neuroses and psychopathies is extremely difficult and hazardous. The majority of these patients never enter mental hospitals. A large percentage of the delinquents, vagabonds, drifters, and other social "failures" probably belong to one or the other groups of psychopathies.

The outward expression assumed by a character disorder often depends on the cultural trends of the environment. Alcoholism does not exist among faithful Mohammedans. It is rare among orthodox Jews, but frequent among the Irish. However, alcoholism is a serious social and medical problem in all American and European countries, and in Russia. In the United States, alcoholics make up 12 per cent of the first admissions to public mental hospitals and they rank high among admissions to general hospitals. Due to their usually deplorable physical and mental condition on admission, they absorb a great proportion of the nursing time without compensating for it with commensurate responses to treatment. Once discharged, they almost invariably return and the cycle of "rehabilitation" starts all over. Compared with the alcoholics, drug addicts and homosexuals constitute a minor problem. Each of these groups makes up a fraction of one per cent of the admissions to public mental hospitals and to the expert it remains a matter of curious concern why the public and the courts of justice react toward them with as much ire and invective as they so often do.

A Psychopathic Personality:

A.F. was sent to N. State Hospital at the age of 35, out of desperation on the part of his family and the various public agencies which for years had tried to help him start a useful life. Each attempt had ended in failure.

On admission A.F., a physically healthy, good looking, but somewhat negligently dressed man, presented himself in a friendly, somewhat condescending way. He quickly established contact with nurses and patients. He proved to be intellectually alert and intelligent, and, with the exception of a certain lack of concern for his situation, his emotional reactions were vivid and commensurate with the topics he discussed. His thinking was clear and coherent and there was no evidence that he suffered from hallucinations or delusions. Concerning his hospitalization, he declared it to be quite unnecessary since he felt neither mentally ill nor in need of any help. On the contrary, he concluded that if people had not interfered so much, he would have been very successful in life. Success, however, was still waiting for him just around the corner. The fact that he had been fired from several jobs or had walked off after a short trial he explained as the result of minor misunderstandings between himself and the boss. He added that people really liked him and that those who had fired him would be glad to have him back, since he was an excellent man with many new ideas. Thus A.F. bragged, lied, and embellished his story, and it remained impossible to reach him, to strike a serious chord in him, to make him reflective. From each discussion with the physician, he emerged like the duck from under the water, unruffled, smiling, and unconcerned.

He was the second son of a fairly successful but detached father with a moderate drinking problem and an affectionate but worrisome mother. His older brother had developed normally, was married, and managed his own business. A sister of his father had been hospitalized on several occasions for psychotic episodes of a manic-depressive disorder.

The patient himself was born without known complications. He appeared precocious in his development, restless, and always curious but quickly dissatisfied. He would attach himself quickly to toys and to other children but would soon lose interest in them. In his relations to his parents he remained unpredictable. As he grew older, frequent fluctuations in his mood became more evident. In school he had no difficulties in mastering the most complicated tasks, but his work was inconsistent, often interrupted by mischievous behavior and truancy. Under much pressure, he finished high school but refused to go any further. The following years were marked by an unending number of apparent attempts to establish himself in a variety of trades. Being a smooth and facile talker, he always found someone who would take him on, but the enchantment would never last more than a few weeks, or at best a few months. Without a sense of personal responsibility or concern for the future and without any lasting attachment to anyone, men or women, A.F. would drift from place to place, occasionally committing minor misdeeds to correct his fortune, and forever writing home for "one more check" so that he could grab "this one tremendous opportunity to strike it rich."

A.F.'s prognosis? A checkup ten years after the hospitalization showed that he had married, was divorced, and still drifting. He had begun to drink. Contacts between him and his aged parents and his brother had practically ceased.

The outstanding feature in A.F.'s character and life is his inadequacy in any given situation. Etiological factors may be seen in his genetic endowment and the emotionally insecure home situation. Dysfunctions in temperament, mood, willpower, and empathy were all evident from the very beginning until the last time we heard of him.

A.F.'s history is typical of a character disorder best designated as inadequate personality.

·V·

Psychoses of Uncertain Etiology

(MANIC-DEPRESSIVE PSYCHOSES, THE SCHIZOPHRENIAS, PARANOID CONDITIONS, INVOLUTIONAL PSYCHOSES.)

Introduction:

In this chapter, mental disorders will be discussed that are clearly different from those dealt with in the preceding pages. Their symptomatologies contain elements that cannot be understood as abnormal variations of behavior since they are not found under normal circumstances. Here, we think of hallucinations and delusions. Other elements, such as alterations in mood, affective contact and thinking, are so grossly distorted as to reach psychotic proportions. Whereas in the case of neuroses and character disorders we can see the emotional development of a person in a certain direction, in all other mental disorders we observe a break in the patient's development, the emergence of something new and foreign, of something which Karl Jaspers and many after him have called a process. A development is something that grows organically, as a seed grows into a flower. A process adversely interrupts a development, as polio-myelitis interrupts the normal development of an extremity. This interruption can be temporary or permanent.

In Chapter VI will be found the disorders in which this process is known, i.e., where a specific agent is recognized as causing the malfunction. In the disorders to be discussed now, the existence of such processes is suspected by many psychiatrists, but, as mentioned earlier, contested by others.

It must be pointed out, however, that clinically these mental disorders of uncertain etiology resemble more closely disorders of toxic and other somatic origins than those we described in the last chapter. Furthermore, hereditary factors are undeniably more significant in their etiologies than they are in all other mental disorders, with the exception of some clearly hereditary chronic brain syndrome, such as Huntington's chorea or certain forms of mental deficiency.

Finally, the often favorable responses to somatic

treatments and the unfavorable responses to psychological treatments differentiate this group of disorders from abnormal reactions and neuroses.

These are the principal reasons for placing the psychoses of unknown etiology, or the functional psychoses, as they are often called, as a separate group in between the abnormal variations of behavior and the brain syndromes. As can be seen on our scale (p. 49) there are no transitions among the three main groups of disorders, but there is considerable overlapping among the three circles constituting the middle group. Indeed, there are patients who show definite mixtures of manic-depressive and schizophrenic symptomatology, and studies in heredity have shown that in the families of these patients pure forms of both disorders can be found.

The involutional psychoses have been classified in various ways. For some psychiatrists paranoid involutional psychoses belong to the group of schizophrenias, for others they constitute a separate entity. The depressive psychoses of the involutional age have been thought to belong to the manic-depressive disorders, but hereditary studies show that they are more often related to the group of schizophrenias. Clinically, they frequently show symptoms belonging to both groups. Thus the arrangement of the circles on our scale becomes meaningful. It must be remembered, however, that future knowledge may necessitate significant changes in this arrangement. The clinical and social importance of these disorders is demonstrated by the fact that they account for well over half of the total admissions to mental hospitals.

MANIC-DEPRESSIVE PSYCHOSES

Definition: Manic-depressive psychoses are characterized by periodic psychotic mood alterations in the form of elations and depressions. Intellectual functions are not affected. The course and pattern of the illness vary and cannot be predicted. The etiology is uncertain; hereditary factors are significant. Somatic treatment is effective in the control of the acute mania and depression. The prognosis for the individual psychotic episode, treated or untreated, is good; that of the ultimate fate of the patient is less so. The most serious complications are suicide during a depression and physical exhaustion in mania.

General Considerations: As name and definition indicate, this disorder has two faces, one laughing and the other crying too much. That the two somehow belong together had been suspected for centuries, but it was Emil Kraepelin who established the final identity of the illness.

The basic dysfunction lies in the area of mood regulation. For this reason manic-depressive psychoses, together with the involutional and possibly other psychotic depressions, have been called affective disorders or affective psychoses. Similar but nonpsychotic mood alterations can be encountered among the psychopathic personalities, and even among normal people there are those who swing back and forth between mild euphoria and mild depression or have a special affinity to one of these moods. Persons with such mood fluctuations are more prone than others to develop manic-depressive disease, but not all manic-depressives have this basic personality structure. The majority of these patients show no psychopathology in between the psychotic episodes.

The prevailing somatotype among people with periodic mood swings is the pyknic or the endomorphic, with some mesomorphic traits. About 60 per cent of all patients with manic-depressive disorders show the former body type. Certain physical diseases, such as arteriosclerosis, hypertension, arthritis, and perhaps diabetes, seem to appear with peculiar frequency in manic-depressive patients.

The dysfunctions in affectivity constitute the fundamental symptoms; the other cardinal manifestations can be understood as their consequences. With different prefixes, they pertain to both manic and depressive phases of the illness. They are: changes in speed and form of thinking, and abnormal facilitation or inhibition of centrifugal functions such as determination, acting, emotional and physical motility. Illusions occur predominantly, delusions frequently, and hallucinations infrequently. Their contents reflect the prevailing mood.

Clinical Syndromes:

The manic phase is characterized by the following principal symptoms: elation, flight of ideas, and extreme restlessness.

A patient going into a manic psychosis will present a clinical picture about as follows: The first sign may be a disturbance in sleep. The patient wakes up early, in excellent spirits, with many plans to be carried out during the day. He walks briskly, keeps busy without getting tired, and talks and jokes more than usual. Initially, his appetite may increase, but soon he will have little desire and less time to eat. He will lose weight. As the psychosis develops, within days or weeks, the euphoria will lead to ecstasy and manic excitement with boundless self-confidence and missionary ideas. Corresponding misinterpretations of reality result. What at first seemed to be purposeful overactivity becomes a hectic and unproductive pseudoactivity.

In his thinking the patient shows flight of ideas, i.e., he speaks rapidly, under great pressure, abandoning scarcely developed thoughts in favor of different ones, triggered by single words, sounds, colors, or objects he hears or observes. Thus, in an attempt to explain how he traveled from his home to the market, a patient may speak of the blue streetcar, the significance of the color blue, the blue sky of California, California's governor (who had become Chief Justice), the Supreme Court, the Last Judgment and the angel food cake he bought in the market. Suddenly, he may interrupt himself, make a most astute remark about the doctor or the nurse in the room and then branch off again in various directions. To the overwhelmed listener the links between the different thoughts always remain recognizable, a significant factor that is missing in the fragmented thought process of the schizophrenic.

While talking the patient will gradually grow more restless, will start doing one thing or another, will shake hands with the physician with the intention of leaving but immediately turn around with more ideas. The doctor's calming efforts or a word of disapproval will trigger a quick change in attitude from friendliness to nastiness. Whereas before he had nothing but praise for his doctor, he now berates him with violent invective, remarkable skill, and often unsurpassable wit.

At this stage, normal inhibitions disappear and the manic becomes very personal in his conversation, sexually provocative, irritable, negligent in dress, manners, and language. Believing himself omnipotent and omniscient, his ideas become grandiose and sometimes delusional. His handwriting is bold and expansive, a few words covering an entire page. Unless hospitalized, the manic may rapidly squander his money by buying incredible quantities of items he hardly needs. He may go into debt by starting a nonsensical business for which he is not equipped. Attempts to restrain him are answered with extreme rage and violence. For his family, the manic patient at large is a nightmare.

However, despite the severity of this condition, it remains possible to establish good emotional contact with the manic patient at least temporarily. He almost never loses his orientation in time and place, although his judgment with regard to his own situation and possibilities suffers severely. In many respects he is overly alert, for instance, in his observations, his ability to draw on memories, and in his skill in debating and argument. If he has delusions or hallucinations they remain fleeting phenomena, which do not gain the significance they have in schizophrenic psychoses.

Without treatment, and sometimes regardless of it, the acute manic phase can last for weeks and months, and since the patients hardly sleep or eat, they can die from exhaustion. Finally, a slowing down of the patient's activities indicates improvement. The ecstasy abates, sleep and appetite improve, weight increases, and thinking becomes normal. Not infrequently the manic phase terminates in a mild and short-lasting depression.

The depressive phase is marked by melancholic mood, inhibition of thinking, and slowing of metabolic functions and movement. Optimism, expansion, facilitation, and high speed, the keywords in the manic phase, are now replaced by their opposites: pessimism, restriction, rigidity, and retardation.

Usually, the first symptoms of a depression are fatigue and apathy, and loss of sleep, appetite, and weight. At this stage many patients appear in the offices of general practitioners complaining of vague physical discomfort, of backaches, headaches, and constipation. The fact that they are primarily depressed is easily overlooked. Symptomatic treatments for their complaints remain ineffective.

As the depression deepens, the patient's mood darkens, the tone of his muscles and skin lessens, he looks sad, feels heavy and slow, and routine tasks cheerfully executed before seem to become great burdens. He quits his job, stays at home, loses interest in his environment, hobbies, food, and sex. Endlessly and painfully his thoughts circle around a very few subjects: his own inadequacy, his past sins, and the hopeless future. Every thought and dream has a pessimistic quality. The slightest mistake made years ago re-emerges as a grossly distorted, haunting memory.

When approached, he is not unfriendly, he listens and is grateful for help even though he believes it to be useless. He speaks with a slow and low voice, but what he says is coherent and understandable in the light of his melancholic mood. For his presumed failures he blames only himself. This contrasts with the attitude of the schizo-phrenic patient who, even when depressed, accuses others of causing his troubles. The depressed readily speaks about his guilt and his anxiety and the deserved punishment he feels is coming. In this respect he may become clearly delusional and take the carpenters' hammering outside the building for a certain sign that everything is being readied for his execution. Occasionally he may hear voices announcing his sins and doom. Although his mind may appear to be dull, a careful observation and some psychological testing will show that his intellectual functions are well preserved. His observations are keen, his memory sharp and his judgment overly critical in some areas invaded by his pessimistic mood.

Being convinced that life can never be happy again and that he is but a burden to those around him, the depressed patient almost invariably harbors suicidal ideas. However, the risk of suicide is not greatest at the nadir of the depression, but at the time when the patient seems slowly to emerge from his depressive apathy and retardation. His thoughts are still deeply pessimistic, but he feels less inhibited in his action. He even is able to muster a faint smile in order to convince his nurse that he is improving. He may ask for the window to be opened to let fresh air come in and then in an unguarded minute he will leap to his death. It is this danger which makes hospitalization almost mandatory.

The depression, too, can last for many months and occasionally for well over a year. Often the first signs of improvement can be noticed on the scale. In both the manic and the depressive phases, gaining of weight is a subtle indicator of a return to normalcy. The patient's mood starts to brighten, first in the evenings; his dreams are encouraging and in the morning he sleeps longer and wakes up more rested. Food begins to taste again, the joy of living returns and gradually pessimism makes room for a cautious optimism. This improvement can develop very slowly, but not infrequently the transition from deep depression to a normal or slightly hypomanic condition comes about very abruptly, often within a single night.

The depressive patient is not always as retarded as described above. Sometimes he is rather restless and excited and one can observe him pacing up and down, ringing his hands in despair and crying. During hospital rounds, he will attempt to follow the physician, voicing endless hypochondriacal complaints, and seeking reassurance and help.

A preponderance of hallucinations and delusions, particularly of a paranoid or at least not clearly depressive content, and signs of emotional detachment are indicative of the presence of schizophrenic elements.

The agitated depressions and the so-called schizo-affective forms belong to that area where the three middle circles on our scale overlap. Their differences manifest themselves not only in the clinical symptomatologies, but also in the responses to treatment.

Course and Prognosis:

Manic-depressive psychoses vary greatly with respect to frequency, alternation, and duration of the individual psychotic phases. Some patients only have depressions; fewer have exclusively manic phases; the majority have both in unpredictable arrangements. Occasionally, there are patients who alternate with clocklike regularity between depressive and manic attacks. The number of attacks any patient may experience during a lifetime varies from one to as many as twenty or more. This great variability of the natural course of the illness renders difficult and precarious any evaluation of what has been hopefully termed preventive therapy.

The first psychotic episode rarely occurs before puberty. The average age of the patient at the onset of the illness lies between fifteen and thirty. According to Vera Norris, the peak for first admissions for manic-depressive disorders to hospitals in London, England, corresponds to the age of fifty-five. In general, then, these psychoses tend to occur later in life than do the schizophrenias. As the patients grow older, depressive phases prevail over manic ones. So far there is no proof that any form of therapy, somatic or psychological, is capable of altering the course of the illness.

Mental deterioration and decisive personality changes are not part of the clinical symptomatology of manic-depressive disorders. The individual depressive and manic phases almost invariably abate spontaneously or much sooner with appropriate treatment. In between psychotic attacks most patients feel and behave normally. However, with increasing age the psychosis-free intervals may become shorter and early arteriosclerotic brain damage can darken the clinical manifestations and the outlook for the patient. Thus, the short-term prognosis for the individual psychotic attack is good, but the long-term prognosis remains dubious.

Etiological Considerations:

While it is true that the precise etiology of manic-depressive psychoses remains uncertain, the author shares the opinion of those who are convinced of the etiological significance of hereditary factors. Mayer-Gross, E. T. Slater, and Roth in *Clinical Psychiatry* state this as follows: "The significance of hereditary factors in the causation of manic-depressive psychoses is established. The mode of inheritance tends to take a dominant form, but gene carriers develop the psychosis in only a minority of cases. The effect of non-genetical factors has therefore also to be taken into account . . ."

Franz Kallman reports 90 per cent concordance for manic-depressive psychoses in identical twins, as against 26 per cent in non-identical twins. Other family risk figures, indicating the chance of one member of the family getting the illness if another has it are: 22 per cent for full siblings, 16 per cent for half-siblings, and 23 per cent for parents.

Contributing factors with respect to etiology can be seen in the endomorphic or pyknic somatotype and the cycloid temperament. This temperament is characterized by frequent mood swings independent of external provocation. Such persons usually are either sociable, good-hearted, and easy going, or elated, humorous, lively, and hot-tempered, or quiet, calm, serious, and gentle.

Are there disease-precipitating factors? This question is difficult to answer. On the surface, it may often be tempting to say that one or another experience triggered a manic or depressive attack. Very minor stimuli of everyday life can serve as such factors. However, it is necessary to remember that to a depressed patient, bemoaning his fancied financial ruin, the announcement that he has just inherited a large sum of money will most probably not terminate his depression. Either he will not believe the messenger or he will shake his head in sadness and say that it will not suffice to satisfy his creditors. To the patient already emerging from his depression, however, the discovery of an extra dollar bill in his pocket may be the occasion of true pleasure and the loss of a dollar bill may be the one event that pushes another into the abyss of a deep psychosis, where undoubtedly he would have ended up anyway. Emotional difficulties are often invoked as being responsible for a psychotic phase, but it may well be that the same difficulties were already the result of the beginning psychosis.

The fact that women are more often affected than men has raised the question of endocrinological factors playing a part in the etiology. As yet, no satisfactory answer has been offered.

With regard to etiology, psychodynamic theories remain without practical value since they can neither be proved nor disproved, as has been pointed out many times in these pages. This does not mean however that psychoanalytical or existential analytical concepts have no value in understanding some of the psychological connections encountered in patients with depressions or manic phases.

Statistical data will be dealt with at the end of this chapter.

Three Manic-Depressive Cousins:

1. *Arthur P.* was one of eleven children, of whom three died in infancy and one during adolescence. Of the seven remaining children, one was a psychopath with very marked mood swings; one, of asthenic body type, was schizophrenic; five were manic-depressive. The parents were cousins and both were hospitalized for manic-depressive psychoses. The mother was of pyknic, the father of asthenic body type. In the ascending, collateral, and descending branches there were an unusual number of persons with manic-depressive illness, with schizophrenia and psychopathy. At the time of his hospitalization, Arthur was described as being of pyknic body type. He suffered from diabetes. As a youngster, he was quiet, dependable, slightly depressed, and very religious. He went to business college, became a traveling salesman, and finally established his own business. At the age of 52, in connection with a financial setback, he developed a severe depression and made a suicide attempt. Within one month, he had improved sufficiently to leave the hospital. One year later he became manic, hardly slept, was euphoric, ordered large quantities of various items for his store, and had to be hospitalized. After two months the manic phase changed into a depressive one. In the following nine years, until his death from a carcinoma, he was hospitalized four more times, mostly for manic attacks. Arthur P. had one daughter who was hospitalized on many occasions for manic and depressive episodes. Her only son, who was

illegitimate, was hospitalized at the age of 22 for an acute manic attack with grandiose behavior, elation, and flight of ideas.

2. *Joshua B.,* a maternal cousin of Arthur P., was one of four children. Both parents were in good mental health, so were his brother and two sisters and their children and grandchildren. Joshua was of pyknic body type and had diabetes. He was a poor learner, lazy, and without scholastic interests. Already, as a child he suffered from marked alternations in mood. At one time he would walk around with a flower in his mouth, singing and happy, and at another he would sit, ruminate, or go into sudden rages. Usually, he appeared to be good-humored, sociable, but prone to hypochondriacal complaints. With his brother he opened a business. At the age of 33, also in connection with financial losses, he became severely depressed. Three years later he married and opened his own business. In this same year he was hospitalized for another depression. In the following years he needed care in four different mental institutions, each time for depression, often triggered by financial setbacks. At the age of 52, he once more entered a mental hospital where he died nine years later of tuberculosis. During these years his mood was mostly depressed, and he remained rigid and unpredictable. Occasionally he would become overactive, euphoric, and clinging.

3. *Isaac G.*'s mother was a sister of Arthur P.'s mother. She married her own cousin, whose mother was a sister of Arthur's maternal grandfather. Isaac was one of thirteen children. Two of these, including Isaac, were manic-

depressive, and five were psychopathic personalities with predominant cyclic mood swings. One healthy brother had a manic-depressive child. Isaac had four children, one of whom was manic-depressive. In school, Isaac was a poor learner. Usually carefree and optimistic, he needed hospitalization as a youngster, probably for a depression. He married at the age of 29, but as husband, father, and businessman he was a complete failure. He squandered his wife's fortune, forged checks, and was a dishonest business partner. At least from the age of 29, he was subject to constant mood alternations. At times he was full of vigor, and had high-flung plans; then he would become anxious, depressed, tremulous, would sit around, talk about suicide and insomnia. Several hospitalizations for depression were necessary. At the age of 57, he suddenly became manic, grandiose, went on a senseless buying spree, made debts, started to drink, and got into trouble with the police. He was hospitalized, found to be manic and of dull normal intelligence. A year later, he ran away from the hospital, but after a few months returned to an outpatient service, this time depressed and dejected. While re-hospitalization was considered, he committed suicide by drowning himself in the nearby river.

THE GROUP OF SCHIZOPHRENIAS

General Considerations:

The psychoses presently constituting the group of schizophrenias represent the greatest challenge in psychiatry today. Almost one quarter of all patients admitted to our mental hospitals for the first time are schizophrenic. Most of them are in the prime of their lives. They tend to stay long, to return after discharge, and many defy all of our treatment methods. Whenever we speak of mental illness, of research in mental illness, of planning for the mentally ill, of the need for a better understanding of the mentally ill on the part of the general population—in short, whenever we speak of the mentally ill as a problem, we think first and foremost of the schizophrenic patient.

It can be assumed that what we call schizophrenia today has existed for many thousands of years. From the earliest available descriptions of mentally ill persons, we can often clearly diagnose schizophrenia. The basic symptoms of the illness must always have been the same. However, it was only in 1896 that the illness was described by Emil Kraepelin as a well-defined entity. Thinking that its two main characteristics were early onset and severe mental deterioration, he gave it the name of *dementia praecox*. He thus contrasted it with diseases leading to mental deterioration in late life and with others of early onset which did not end in mental deterioration, such as the manic-depressive psychoses.

Eugen Bleuler, in Switzerland, basically accepting the description and subdivision of the illness, took issue with Kraepelin's pessimistic statements as to its course and outcome. He noticed that the disease often appears relatively late in life and that one third of the schizophrenic patients recover spontaneously and another third improve sufficiently to be released from the hospital. He emphasized as characteristic the peculiar condition of the

illness that seems to permit the patient to live simultaneously in two worlds, the world of reality and a world
of delusions. For this reason, he proposed the term
schizophrenia, later generally accepted (from the Greek
words ΣΧΙΖΕΙΥ, to split, and ΦΡΗΟ, mind). His mono-
graph *Dementia Praecox or the Group of Schizophrenias*
(1911) has remained the classic description of the illness,
its possible etiological factors, and its management. Today,
it is almost as modern as it was fifty years ago.

Emil Kraepelin's original concept of dementia praecox
was widened by Eugen Bleuler to encompass clinical
syndromes which Kraepelin probably would not have
considered as belonging to dementia praecox. In subsequent decades the disease concept underwent some further
modifications. For some, paranoid states and paranoia
were considered to belong to the group of schizophrenias;
at other times they were considered not to belong. The
borderland between manic-depressive and schizophrenic
psychoses was claimed alternatively by the two camps.
This is well reflected in the records of patients who were
repeatedly admitted to the same hospital between the
years 1900 and 1950. The descriptions of the symptoms
were always identical, but the labels shifted.

With the designation "group of schizophrenias" Bleuler
intended to indicate not only that the illness assumes
different clinical syndromes, held together only by the
basic schizophrenic symptoms, but also that the etiology is
most probably multifactorial. It is unfortunate that this
was often forgotten. Psychiatrists started to speak of
"schizophrenia" as if it were one disease showing different
manifestations. They endeavored to find "the cause" and

since some sought it in biological and others in psychological processes two hostile camps were formed. Bleuler
himself was less arbitrary and much wiser than many of his
followers, who perhaps had never read his book. Finally
the term "schizophrenic reaction" appeared, attempting to
sneak through the back door a prematurely etiological, i.e.,
psychogenic definition. Thus it was assumed that the ego
of a person who as a child had undergone specific
traumatic experiences would, under severe stress, build up
defense mechanisms in the form of schizophrenic syndromes. This is an unproven and probably unwarranted
theory on which the author will not elaborate further.

Of late, a retrograde movement has been taking place.
For some years European authors, particularly G. Langfeld
in Norway, have advocated the separation of true or
nuclear schizophrenic psychoses from schizophrenia-like
psychoses. The first group would fall under a disease
concept similar to Kraepelin's and would comprise
psychoses of early onset and bad outcome. Among the
second group would be classified all those psychoses of
varying onset ending in recovery. Among the latter, we
would find some toxic, infectious, or reactive psychoses
which at least temporarily have all the clinical earmarks of
schizophrenia. Bleuler's son, Manfred Bleuler, has adopted
this viewpoint and speaks of schizophrenia, symptomatic
schizophrenia, and schizophrenic reactions.

All this is indicative of attempts to solve the complex
problem of schizophrenia. One fact seems to be clear: in
the face of the diversity of the clinical phenomena it is

almost impossible to think of the schizophrenias in terms
of a uniform disease process with a single causative factor.
In this text, we will follow Eugen Bleuler's original
concept and once again speak of the group of schizophrenias, leaving open the question of the uniformity and
causation of this illness, which for the time being remains
as enigmatic as it is terrible.

Definition: Presently, in American psychiatry, the group
of schizophrenias comprises six syndromes or subgroups:
simple schizophrenia, hebephrenia, catatonia, paranoid
schizophrenia, schizo-affective schizophrenia, and undifferentiated schizophrenia All syndromes have certain primary
symptoms in common; i.e., specific changes in affectivity,
in the thought process, and in volition. Accessory
symptoms, such as delusions and hallucinations, catatonic
stupor, confusion, and mannerisms, may be present at
times and to different degrees and distributions in the
various subgroups. The personality of the patient under-
goes a decisive and characteristic change which can always
be detected on close scrutiny. The course of the illness is
phasic. It manifests itself as a single attack or as multiple
acute psychotic episodes, or it can be chronic, leading to a
severe personality disintegration. The etiology is uncertain
but is most probably multifactorial. Consciousness is clear,
sensory and intellectual faculties in themselves are not
affected, but the proper use of them almost invariably is.

SUBGROUPS

Commentary: The individual subgroups will be described below. They are determined by the predominant accessory symptoms. Thus a schizophrenic who suffers primarily from persecutory or paranoid delusions and hallucinations will be called paranoid; another, mostly mute, rigid and tense, is called catatonic. This does not exclude the fact that the paranoid patient occasionally refuses to speak or to move out of the corner where he stands for hours, watching silently, nor that the catatonic may harbor paranoid ideas. Paranoid delusions are found in all mental disorders. The characteristic is not the presence of the symptoms but the circumstances under which they appear and the manner in which they are explained and maintained. Shifts from one subtype to another can be observed during a single psychotic episode or in chronic cases over a period of years.

PRIMARY SYMPTOMS

The diagnosis of schizophrenia cannot be made in the absence of all of the primary symptoms. This is an important point, deserving close attention. According to the present definition of the illness, no amount of hallucinations or delusions and no psychodynamic constellation, as convincing as it may appear, can serve as basis for the diagnosis.

The changes in affectivity are the most characteristic features in schizophrenia. Lending a peculiar flavor to all other symptoms and to the entire personality of the patient, they alone permit a convincing diagnosis. We distinguish changes in affective contact and in emotional responses.

AFFECTIVE CONTACT

We call man's ability to establish an emotional relationship or involvement with other persons, objects, or ideas affective contact. What has previously been termed empathy is part of this emotional involvement. A normal human being is emotionally involved in a wide area: in people, deceased and living; in objects, far and near; and in thoughts, past and present. These form his own world, his sphere of interest, and it is the affectivity he has invested in them that truly makes it his personal world. In schizophrenia this sphere of interest, this affective involvement seems to shrink. Gradually the patient loses interest in his environment and contact with those around him. He appears to be impenetrable, living behind a glass wall, or in a vacuum. Emotional contact involves a certain trust, openness and willingness to listen. Emotional contact is like an invisible fabric stretched out between two persons, and if it is good, it will endure a certain amount of wear and tear, arguments, and disappointments. In schizophrenia the fabric is brittle, trust has been replaced by uncertainty and suspiciousness. The affective bridge between the schizophrenic and his former world has broken down. These affective changes are difficult to describe, but to the sensitive diagnostician they are revealed in almost everything a schizophrenic person does or says. They are responsible for the oddities and estrangement which we do not find in any other mental illness. The isolation and withdrawal of the schizophrenic we call autism. In its extreme forms the patient is absorbed in a world·of fantasies, delusions, and hallucinations, and pays little or no attention to his surroundings.

EMOTIONAL RESPONSE

The changes in the emotional responses are intimately related to the changes in affective contact. There is an incongruity between affect and thought, spoken word or action. Thus a serious event can be reported with laughter or an enigmatic smile which seems to be completely out of place. More often, we find a blunting of all affective responses. Whatever the patient says is said in the same monotonous voice, accompanied by a flat, unmodulated facial expression. This increases the impression of coldness and uneasiness one often experiences in the presence of schizophrenics.

THOUGHT PROCESS

The disturbances in the thought process further contribute to the splitting up and disintegration of the personality of the schizophrenic. In listening to a manic patient, we are, with some effort, always able to follow his flight of ideas. We can understand him. With the schizophrenic, this often becomes difficult or impossible. In his thinking, he is incoherent, fragmented, and illogical. In the middle of a sentence he may break off one train of thought and pursue another apparently unconnected with the first. If there are connections at all, they must be unconscious, inexplainable to both the speaker and the listener. Where the manic might say: "I rode in this blue bus, blue means hope, you know, knowledge is so important ..." the schizophrenic could say: "I rode this blue bus, my mother never wanted me to cry, but we are all small when it comes to eternity ..." Listening to the first sentence we may smile, but hearing the second, which really is not a sentence any more, we can only shake our head in bewilderment, because we cannot even guess what prompted its sequence.

The thinking is not focused; it is besides the point and illogical, emphasizing the detail instead of what is important; it is concrete where it should be abstract, and abstract where it should be concrete. The patient himself is not aware of such changes; he believes he is clear and logical and tends to become angry if challenged.

Other changes in the thinking process concern sudden blocking. Particularly the catatonic patient is apt to stop talking in the middle of a sentence. After a while, he may continue to speak, but about something else. Other patients complain that they cannot concentrate, that they are not masters of their own thoughts, that foreign thoughts are being put into their head while their own thoughts are pulled out; or they complain that thoughts are rushing through their mind at such a speed that they become confused. The patients are usually aware of such changes, but they attribute them to mostly unfriendly external influences.

Changes in thinking are not always obvious. In paranoid schizophrenics one has to listen carefully in order to detect them, whereas in hebephrenic patients, the listener may be overwhelmed by a complete word salad.

Many patients speak coherently and logically about emotionally indifferent topics, but become fragmented and illogical when discussing problematic and emotionally charged matters.

VOLITION

The changes in volition can be summarized by the terms ambivalence and negativism. Here, too, the disturbances in the patient's affectivity play an important part. A person who feels simultaneously attracted and repelled by another person, object, action, or thought is called ambivalent. In schizophrenia, ambivalence can become so pronounced that it freezes all action and decision-making. The patient cannot make up his mind about how he feels, what he wants to do, what he should say. Thus throughout an entire interview a schizophrenic may repeat: "It can be this way and it can be the other way," or "I am not sure how I feel, you are the doctor, you ought to know." Being unable to decide whether or not he should leave the room or participate in a game, a patient may stand stiffly in a corner until the game is over.

Negativism is another aspect of impaired volition. The catatonic patient demonstrates it when he goes backward if asked to come forward, when he shrugs at the outstretched hand of the doctor and refuses to participate in any activity. What puts the stamp of negativism on such behavior is the seeming lack of motivation. If one sits down next to a depressed patient in order to comfort him, he will either not move or will turn toward you; the schizophrenic automatically moves or turns away. The one shows need for affective warmth, the other is afraid of it, avoids it, is negativistic. Negativism expresses itself in attitudes, in speech, and in writing. It can be observed in all schizophrenics and is always a puzzling and chilling experience for the unprepared who approaches the patient with open hands.

ACCESSORY SYMPTOMS

Illusions and delusions are seldom missing in schizophrenia. An illusion is a false interpretation of something seen, heard, or felt. For example, a curtain moved by a current of air can suddenly be interpreted as a man moving in a dark corner. Often the first symptoms of schizophrenia are misconceptions of the world around. To the patient the faces of parents and other people may suddenly seem to be distorted and to express disgust or hate. What had been familiar for years becomes unfamiliar and strange. Actually, such misconceptions may already be delusions, i.e., false beliefs that have no factual basis in reality. The schizophrenic may believe that he is Napoleon or God or that the Freemasons have decided to eliminate him. Delusions of persecution and grandeur are found most frequently. In paranoid schizophrenics, delusions form a more or less elaborated system in which the patient is the center of attention.

Hallucinations are sensory perceptions without any physical substance. Voices are heard in a soundless room or in an open area where nobody is around except the patient. Faces appear on the wall of a room or suspended in mid air, strange odors are perceived, and at night the patient may feel that he is being touched, influenced with electricity, or that someone is playing with his sexual organs. In most cases delusions precede hallucinations, but the latter reinforce them. Sometimes they are contradictory, thus reflecting the ambivalence and fragmentation of the schizophrenic personality.

In schizophrenia, auditory hallucinations ("voices") predominate; visual hallucinations are relatively rare. What distinguishes the schizophrenic voices from those heard in an alcoholic delirium, for instance, is the fact that they are heard in the absence of a clouded consciousness or of organic brain deterioration. The patient may hear voices while quietly reading a book. Unlike the alcoholic, he will probably not show any particular reaction to them. When he hears voices for the very first time, he somehow takes them for granted. Further, whereas the alcoholic often "accidentally overhears" other people talking about him, the schizophrenic is spoken to directly. There is nothing accidental about this and usually nothing playful. The alcoholic readily talks about his hallucinations, jokingly and angrily and with a speck of skepticism. The schizophrenic rarely questions the reality of the voices, and he does not like to talk about them. In the more chronic stage of the illness, the voices may assume a more benign character and often the patients consider them to be good company.

Another important accessory symptom is the catatonic stupor, during which the patient appears frozen in a certain attitude or position. He may not even swallow his saliva, which will drool out of his half open mouth or accumulate behind his tightly clenched teeth and lips. This facade of motionless rigidity may hide an acutely observing mind, though one plagued by delusions and hallucinations.

The Subgroups:

Simple Schizophrenia is characterized by the presence of primary symptoms only. Delusions and hallucinations do not occur, or if they do, they remain fleeting phenomena. The illness develops insidiously over a period of years, invariably leading to a severe disintegration of the personality.

The most striking feature of the illness is a gradual loss of affectivity, activity, and interest. Previously spirited persons become content to spend hours, then days, and finally years in complete idleness. They neglect their appearance, their habits, they withdraw from all contact with friends and gradually sink into social, intellectual, and emotional oblivion. In conversation, they are bland, unmoved by prodding, and their thought disorder can be detected only in the illogical arguments they use to explain their behavior. They completely lack insight into their failure.

Sometimes in the early stages of the illness a patient may commit an isolated crime which stands out because of the peculiar callousness and detachment with which it was accomplished. Or the lack of empathy and contact may manifest itself in fraudulent or otherwise irresponsible behavior in business or marriage. Since, for a time at least, their intellectual faculties are not distorted by the changes in affectivity, these people can become serious social problems.

Catatonic Schizophrenia contrasts sharply with the simple form. All primary symptoms are found and a host of accessory ones—the outstanding of them, catatonic attitudes and stupor. For the most part, the illness strikes suddenly, although to the observant family prodromal signs become apparent over a period of months. Within a few days, the patient may changes his entire behavior. He becomes suspicious, seclusive, and negativistic, and refuses to leave the house. He finally stops eating, becomes mute, and for hours stands, sits, or lies around in uncomfortable positions. Odd mannerisms, sudden grimaces and movements may indicate that the patient hallucinates. Attempts to converse with him are met with hostile glances, and insistence may bring about sudden attacks of extreme violence. Unexpectedly, the mutism can be interrupted by abrupt remarks which show the double registration so typical for schizophrenia; for example, when the patient is delusional or grandiose, but simultaneously knows exactly what is going on and who he really is. Thus, a mute and tense patient suddenly points at Dr. Smith and in horror yells, "You are not Dr. Smith, you are the devil," but then proceeds to let Dr. Smith give him an injection without offering the slightest resistance. This cannot be predicted, however.

Catatonic rigidity can last for days, months, or years. It can alternate with periods of catatonic agitation or with times of relative quiescence. The illness can come over the patient like a storm, shake him to the roots, and leave him little altered, with no precise memory of what has happened. Or it can rapidly lead to a chronic stage with severe personality disintegration and untidiness in all habits.

Hebephrenic Schizophrenia is the most colorful and, to the observer, perhaps the most tragic schizophrenic syndrome. All primary symptoms are maximally developed and with them a great variety of ever-changing accessory symptoms, such as auditory, visual, and tactile hallucinations, weird delusions, mannerisms, and abstruse, overactive behavior. In general, the illness quickly develops toward a severe personality disintegration.

Hebephrenia, as the name indicates, has its onset in adolescence. A young girl, originally quiet and diligent, either progressively or quite suddenly changes into a restless, inattentive, giggling, and facetious little person. Vainly, parents and teachers try to reason with her. Schooling has to be terminated. At a number of jobs the girl does not concentrate, does not learn, and, worst of all, cannot behave. Her speech becomes rambling and fragmented, her laughter silly, and in order to break through her growing isolation and to reach others, she behaves like a clown. This last remark is obviously interpretation, but one that comes easily. Increasingly odd and unpredictable behavior—often in response to hallucinations and delusions—overactivity alternating with apathy, moodiness, sexual promiscuity, and possible minor delinquency, soon make hospitalization mandatory.

At this stage, these patients are often serious management problems. It is difficult to reach them. They readily get into trouble with other patients, although, unlike the psychopath, they remain at the periphery of any ward population. Hypochondriacal complaints, outbursts of anger or laughter over preposterous hallucinations, delusions of grandeur, inconsistencies, and unreliability complete the picture. The course of the illness may be phasic, with exacerbations and periods of apparent reintegration, but as the years advance, the patient loses much of his overactivity and becomes more apathetic, but remains hallucinated, delusional, and silly.

Paranoid Schizophrenia is the opposite of hebephrenia in almost every respect. Where the hebephrenic is silly, flighty, and inconsistent, the paranoid is serious, logical, and persistent. The paranoid schizophrenic shows a minimum of primary symptoms, and of the accessory ones, delusions of persecution are predominant. Usually his personality remains well preserved, and socially he may function quite appropriately until his delusions interfere with his activities.

Of all the schizophrenic syndromes, the paranoid has the latest onset. Insidiously, it tends to develop in persons with a good work record and an outwardly stable, somewhat rigid personality. The first symptoms may be a gradual withdrawal from co-workers, increased aloofness, and here and there a suspicious frown or look. The person starts to observe. Soon he finds what he is looking for: when he comes to his office desk in the morning, he can tell that someone has been looking into his drawer. When he passes others, he notices that their conversation stops, or that they change the topic. To him, it is obvious that they talk about him, that they know what is going on, whereas he does not. He decides to ask a direct question, but nobody seems to understand, "naturally." "Accidentally" he overhears that the main office conducts a general inspection and in the newspaper his attention is drawn, for the first time, to the daily report of a committee on anti-government activities. Looking out of the window, he notices a car standing at the corner; it was not there yesterday. At night, the telephone rings, but all he hears is some cautious breathing, a faint rustle, and laughter. By now the patient feels cornered and evidence of a plot against him multiplies: people in the street spit when they see him, remarks are being made about him over the radio and on television; the coffee tastes peculiar; the room and even the bed are wired. In his desperation, he goes to his boss, to the police, to the FBI, and for his own protection he may carry a gun. By now everybody except the patient himself realizes that he is mentally ill and in need of hospitalization.

In the hospital the patient is tense, hostile, aloof, and suspicious. He tends to be somewhat formal, cautious; contact is tenuous, but his emotional reactions correspond to the content of his thoughts. His first statement is that he did not come to the hospital, that he was brought. His speech is coherent, and, as a matter of fact, is well focused. With seeming logic, he speaks about the "plot," the persecution, the interferences, and it is only when one tries to point out some inconsistencies and the unreasonable-ness of his assumptions that the thought disorder becomes increasingly apparent. Often, the patients feel safe and relaxed in the hospital and for hours one can converse with them on neutral subjects, politics, art, and travel, and will find them pleasant, witty, and coherent.

Not all paranoid schizophrenics develop in such a rather consequential fashion. Delusions can be much more scattered in appearance and content, hallucinations can be more or less prominent, and there may be some catatonic features. What is essential is the predominant theme of suspiciousness, of malevolent interference, and, underlying this, ideas of increased self-importance.

Paranoid schizophrenia can run a steady course toward progressive personality disintegration, during which the initial inner logic of the system breaks down and hallucinations and delusions become more and more fantastic and inconsistent with the original master plan. Thinking becomes grossly fragmented and autism increases. However, some paranoids preserve their delusional systems as well as their personality for many decades and manage to function socially. There are also a good number of these patients who recover spontaneously, or after treatment for a few months or years, and return to their previous, probably somewhat restricted, life.

Undifferentiated Schizophrenia comprises those schizophrenic syndromes which lack any of the outstanding characteristics mentioned above. Primary and accessory symptoms are present in varying constellations and intensity. The onset can be early or late, insidious or rapid, and the course cannot be predicted. In their chronic stages many of the other syndromes develop into the undifferentiated forms of schizophrenia, constituting a large proportion of the population of mental hospitals.

Schizo-affective Schizophrenia in many ways resembles the syndromes of manic-depressive psychosis. Often the patients are of the endomorphic body type. Their original personality differs from those of the other schizophrenics inasmuch as they tend to be quite sociable and outgoing, but subject to mood swings. Their schizophrenic psychoses are marked by affective changes in the sense of depression or elation, with remnants of good emotional contact. However, the thought process shows the earmarks of fragmentation, and there are delusions and hallucinations in the absence of marked depression or excitement. The course is phasic, resembling that of manic-depressive psychoses. For the most part these patients recover spontaneously, or respond to treatment better than any other schizophrenics, and between the psychotic episodes they function well socially. Their personalities do not show a strong tendency toward disintegration as seen in other subtypes.

Paranoid Conditions and Paranoia:

As mentioned earlier, there has been considerable controversy over the classification of certain paranoid conditions that appear to differ from paranoid schizo-phrenia with regard to specific psychopathology, social functioning, and outcome. Some psychiatrists placed them into separate categories, others considered them to belong to the manic-depressive psychoses, and many thought, and still think, that they belong to the group of schizophrenias. Without entering this debate, the author, with due reservations, will include these rare conditions in this chapter on schizophrenia.

PARANOID CONDITIONS

Paranoid conditions have been described as clinical syndromes manifested by paranoid delusions, centered around a
specific psychologically sensitive topic with marked affective changes; thought disturbances, and secondary symptoms, except for persecutory delusions, are not present.
The illness does not lead to a general personality disintegration and often the patient continues to function
socially. In many cases, spontaneous resolution of the
persecutory ideas occurs within a few months. Paranoid
conditions assume an intermediate position between paranoid schizophrenia and paranoia. The delusions are neither
as scattered and all-pervasive as in paranoid schizophrenia,
nor as systematized and fanatically adhered to as in
paranoia.

PARANOIA

In paranoia the delusions form a tight system of ideas,
based on wrong premises, but logical in itself. The
personality is well preserved. The paranoid system often
takes its origin in a falsely interpreted actual occurrence
and then grows, slowly but inexorably. The nuclear idea is
deeply embedded in the person's character structure.
Often these patients are convinced that they have a
specific mission, and with incredible skill, intelligence, and
tenacity, they can pursue their cause in courts of law,
gather followers, and get the support of newspapers.

Paranoia and paranoid conditions have their onset relatively late in life, but whereas the latter may fade away, paranoia does not. The delusions finally destroy the patient in one way or another—a process demonstrated many times in history by religious, political, and other fanatics.

Not many cases of true paranoia have been described in literature. Karl Kahlbaum, who invented the name, and Emil Kraepelin thought they had a number of such patients, and felt justified in placing them in a separate category. However, a later re-evaluation of these original cases showed that many of them had subsequently become schizophrenic. Thus in the presence of all paranoid conditions we always have to consider the possibility that we are dealing with mild or atypical forms of schizophrenia.

COURSE

Course and Outcome:

Predominantly, the schizophrenias are chronic but phasic diseases, showing marked variations in course and outcome. E. Bleuler found that about one third of all schizophrenic patients recover, another third improve considerably, and the last third remain in hospitals or in need of some other permanent care. In spite of all our modern treatment modalities this basic rule still applies. M. Bleuler has made a further differentiation between simple and undulant courses and, in each of these, among those leading to defect and others ending in dementia. By the term "dementia" we understand a degree of deterioration of the entire personality, including intellectual faculties, that permanently precludes independent social function. "Defect" means a condition that permits independent living and working, although the illness has left a distinctive mark on the personality in the sense of an emotional impoverishment and general restriction. Remnants of primary as well as secondary symptoms can often be found in these patients, who otherwise may perform fairly complicated tasks, at a level slightly below their premorbid one.

In the simple courses the illness, acutely or slowly but without remission, leads to dementia in about 25 per cent of the cases, and to defect in another 10 per cent. In the undulant forms, the disease process is characterized by partial or complete remission alternating with exacerbations ending in dementia in 5 percent, and in defect in 35 per cent of the cases. Finally, in another 30 per cent of the patients, one or several acute psychotic episodes are followed by remission without detectable defect. According to M. Bleuler, hereditary or other somatic factors (endocrinological ones, for instance) decide the course of the illness, whereas treatment and environment determine the final condition of the patient. In other words, although the most elaborate therapeutic program cannot prevent some patients from rapidly sinking into complete oblivion, many who would do the same if they were left alone can be helped to remain more active and interested in the realities of this world.

PROGNOSIS

Some factors seem to be related to course and outcome and are of prognostic value. They involve somatic and psychological criteria often appearing in established patterns and are easily detected. The following are considered to be favorable prognostic signs: an endomorphic somatotype, an outgoing, warm, and affectionate personality, a stable work record, rapid and late onset of the illness, obvious precipitating factors, remnants of good emotional contact, and affective mood fluctuations, or delirious confusion during the psychosis. Unfavorable signs: an ectomorphic body type, a schizoid personality characterized by shyness, seclusiveness and aloofness, an erratic work record, early and insidious onset of the illness without any evidence of precipitating factors such as physical illness, childbirth or serious emotional stress, and the absence of any affective modulations in the psychopathology.

In general, the simple and the hebephrenic subtypes of schizophrenia have an unfavorable prognosis, whereas the outlook for catatonic, paranoid, and particularly the schizo-affective syndromes is better.

Etiological Considerations:

Keeping in mind that the etiology or etiologies of schizophrenia are still uncertain, those factors which are likely to be or to become significant and those others which may be of a disease-precipitating nature have to be discussed. It must be understood that an etiological factor is one without which the illness cannot appear. This rule does not apply to the precipitating factors.

HEREDITY

There can be little doubt that heredity plays an important role in the etiology of schizophrenia. This has always been maintained by most European psychiatrists and is being increasingly accepted in the United States.

Wherever reliable data are available, the incidence of schizophrenia in the general populations throughout the world is 0.8 to 1.0 per cent. Investigations of relatives of schizophrenics have shown the following pattern: For second degree relatives the risk of becoming schizophrenic is about 3 per cent. For first degree relatives it is 10 per cent. If both parents are schizophrenic, their children face an expectancy of 40 per cent. Naturally, as in all hereditary investigations of man, twin studies are of particular interest. In schizophrenia, fraternal or heterozygous twins have an expectancy for the illness of about 11 per cent, whereas for identical or monozygotic twins it rises sharply to between 50 and 80 per cent, according to a variety of investigations. Identical twins reared together have a higher expectancy than identical twins reared apart (91 and 77 per cent respectively, according to Kallman).

That heredity plays an important role in the etiology of schizophrenia few doubt. However, if schizophrenia were a purely genetic illness we would have to expect a concordance rate for monozygotic twins of 100 per cent.

Other factors must also play a role. Here it is of interest that among non-identical twins, the one who develops schizophrenia is lighter, weaker and shorter at birth, has more complications at birth (including asphyxia), shows more neurologic signs of brain damage, and, in childhood, displays more characteristics typical of the pre-psychotic personality of the schizophrenic, such as "neurotic" behavior, shyness, submissiveness, greater sensitivity, dependency and seriousness. In general, the non-schizophrenic twin shows a greater variety of abnormal behavior than would be expected normally. Present research is focusing much attention on this complicated question: What are the genetic and what the environmental factors in the genesis of schizophrenia?

In summary we may say that a genetic factor in the transmission of schizophrenia does exist; that we do not yet know the mode of this transmission, but that it is most likely polygenic in nature (as opposed to a simple dominant or recessive genetic factor), and that intra-uterine complications, as well as complications at birth, play an important role. Evidently this points to the necessity of giving the greatest possible care to pregnant women who are, or whose husbands are, schizophrenic.

CONSTITUTION

Two thirds of all schizophrenics are found to be of an ectomorphic body type often mixed with mesomorphic elements. The ectomorphic somatotype has been associated with rather specific personality traits, subsumed under the name of schizoid personality. This personality, which has been described earlier, is characterized by the simultaneous presence of often sharply contrasting qualities. Thus, schizoid persons can be emotionally dull in one area and oversensitive in another, or overly quiet and highly excitable, serious and also eccentric, good-hearted and aloof. This personality is found significantly more often among persons who later become schizophrenic than it is in the general population.

BIOCHEMICAL CONCEPTS

To date no anatomic changes have been demonstrated in the brains of schizophrenics. Therefore, research into organic concepts is based on the assumption that the clinical picture of schizophrenia results from abnormal physiological processes affecting the brain.

About 20 years ago Smythies and Osmond suggested that schizophrenia might be the result of some toxin in the body, and that this toxin could derive from a genetically defective metabolism of epinephrine. Epinephrine is a biogenic amine, related to adrenaline, that plays an important part in brain functions. Among a variety of possibilities with regard to a faulty epinephrine metabolism, it has been postulated that at one stage of this metabolism a hallucinogenic substance, chemically related to mescaline, can be produced.

At this point it must be inserted that the use and abuse of such substances as mescaline and LSD 25 have greatly stimulated and enhanced biochemical studies into the nature of schizophrenia. When ingested, these and similar substances bring about psychotic states resembling in many ways the clinical symptoms of schizophrenia, and most of them are cousins of chemical compounds present in the human body and instrumental in the proper functioning of brain activities.

The next question is: Where in the brain do these substances play their part? One of the principal investigators in this field has been Robert G. Heath of Tulane University. Animal experiments show that lesions in certain areas of the frontal brain and in the deep structures of the midbrain alter or lower awareness and emotional feelings and expressions in such a way as to resemble those seen in schizophrenia. Very delicate electrodes placed deeply in the frontal (septal) parts of the brain record abnormal electrical discharges during psychotic behavior. They can be graphically recorded in an electro-encephalogram. Such findings are not confined to schizophrenia, but are equally present in vascular diseases of the brain during drug-induced and other episodic psychoses. Their intensity changes with the course of the psychoses.

It has also been found that relationships exist between sensory perception and psychotic states. Monkeys deprived of certain types of sensory input in critical stages of their early development, exhibit irreversible gross behavioral manifestations resembling psychotic states. Here part of the cerebellum, the deep seated centers in the midbrain and the forebrain, is involved, and the critical sites for the faulty functioning, i.e., the transmission of nerve impulses, are the synapses. (See Fig. 1, Chap. II.) Responsible for the transmission of the impulses are transmitter amines, such as epinephrine and serotonine. It can be assumed that in psychotic states we deal either with a faulty metabolism of these substances or with other interferences in the transmission of them. In some experiments, abnormal endproducts of a faulty amine metabolism have been found in the urine of schizophrenics more often than in normal control subjects.

That these are not merely idle speculations seems to be born out by the fact that drugs effective in schizophrenic and manic-depressive disease, such as Thorazine and Tofranil (i.e., phenothiazines and their antidepressive derivatives), as well as the non-phenothiazine antidepressives, Parnate, Nardil and Marplan (monoaminooxidase inhibitors) do affect nerve impulse transmission at the synapses involving epinephrine and serotonine, which in turn are related to psychominetic drugs, particularly mescaline and tryptamine derivatives.

Furthermore it is of interest that only those phenothiazines are therapeutically effective which produce side effects known as parkinsonism, a neurological disease based on pathological alterations in certain deep seated centers in the brain. Thus we have the following equations: Phenothiazines affect dopamine metabolism. (Dopamine is another substance of the metabolic chain involving adrenalin-epinephrine and serotonine and tryptamine.) In parkinsonism we find low dopamine levels in certain so-called extrapyramidal centers of the brain. Parkinsonism is now effectively ameliorated by the administration of L-Dopa. L-Dopa produces psychotic symptoms resembling those of schizophrenia.

As interesting and scientifically promising as all this is, it must be stressed that to date we do not have any central theory that pulls together these various findings and ideas.

SOCIAL AND CULTURAL CONCEPTS

One of the central themes in the study of schizophrenia is the problem of communication and relatedness. The schizophrenic is an extremely isolated and lonely person. Unquestionably, communicating and relating with others is learned in earliest childhood within the setting of the family. The question then arises, what went wrong and why?

In an attempt to answer this we must consider (1) genetic factors which may determine response dispositions as one aspect of a person's basic temperament; (2) social class in the sense of representing certain specific ways of thinking, feeling and expression; (3) intrafamily communications, i.e., the way various members of a family deal with or respond to each other. Research has shown that families with one schizophrenic member have more other, non-schizophrenic, communication abnormalities than other families. Most likely these three factors interact closely with each other.

Although schizophrenia is found in all social settings, the greatest incidence is in the lowest social class levels. Why this is so is not well understood. According to Melvin Kohn* of NIMH there are three major theories:

1. The drift hypothesis: Schizophrenics or their parents are in the lower class because they cannot perform adequately in any given society, and therefore cannot maintain a higher social status. However, statistics do not seem to support this theory as the only explanation.

*Medcomsympos. (Pfizer), 1971.

2. The greater incidence of schizophrenia in the lowest social class has nothing to do with class itself but rather with social isolation, social integration, or the lack of it, discrepancies between aspirations and achievement and minority positions. Such conditions are favored in lower social class levels.

3. Conditions of life built into lower social class positions are conducive to the development of schizophrenia. Stress is more prevalent in lower social class, views are held with greater rigidity, the orientational systems are more limited, people are more fearful and distrustful, are more fatalistic and lacking in self confidence. Here, again, genetic factors may play an important part. This third theory seems to be the most promising one, but much further research is necessary to reach scientifically more satisfying conclusions that permit their integration with those of the biochemists.

ANALYTICAL CONCEPTS

If the propositions discussed above are relevant, it still remains to be explained how the genetic predisposition, the biochemical findings and the environmental stresses, together or separately, create the specific symptomatology of schizophrenia. Analytically oriented psychiatry attempts to give an answer.

Although Sigmund Freud himself did not think that psychoanalytical theory and therapy were applicable to entities such as schizophrenia and manic-depressive disease, he nevertheless pointed for example at the link between guilt and psychotic paranoid thinking. Many of his followers have tried to understand schizophrenia purely in terms of psychoanalytical concepts. This author has serious doubts that this is possible, and to him the results of psychoanalytical therapy alone in cases of schizophrenia do not look promising. However, here again the last word has certainly not been spoken.

Viewing schizophrenia from an analytical vantage point, Otto A. Will* gives the following brief summary of the most important symptoms and their possible psychological origin.

Schizophrenic symptoms appearing in later life are the result of unresolved and uncorrected conflicts in early infancy learning patterns.

The schizophrenic has a great need, but an equally great fear of attaching himself to others. This can be the result of a failure to develop trusting attachments in early life. Concomitant with this is a constant fear of threatened loss and separation.

The schizophrenic's preference for using symbols in his speech and behavior are thought of as a mode of defense and cryptic communication developed within the first year of life.

Frequently the schizophrenic has a rather shaky image of his own body, doubts that some parts of it belong to him, or believes that his body is possessed by evil elements. This would be part of his early inability to trust others and thus develop trust in himself.

Cardinal symptoms of schizophrenia are dissociation and fragmentation manifested in speech and expression of feelings. The schizophrenic blocks out awareness of certain aspects of his own development and thus maintains a certain emotional equilibrium, defends himself against

*Medcomsympos. (Pfizer), 1971.

threatening intrusions. He has become aware in his childhood that some sorts of behavior are unacceptable, and his cautious avoidance of such behavior works well until he is forced under particular stress to expose himself more fully. If this happens he panics and develops symptoms of schizophrenia.

The frequently observed withdrawal and somnolent detachment of the schizophrenic are seen as a return to defense mechanisms in childhood. In an unpleasant anxiety-creating situation, the infant cannot destroy, attack or run away, but he can withdraw.

Anxiety and feeling of impending panic are universal in schizophrenia and are reminiscent of the child's fear of breaking down, of losing his sense of being a fully integrated personality.

Like many children, schizophrenics are often full of fear of their own potential destructiveness and aggression. They conceive themselves as being evil.

Hallucinations and delusions are conceived as symbolic processes of early, poorly integrated experiences.

These analytical concepts are interesting, if not always wholly convincing. They and genetic and cultural factors are not necessarily mutually exclusive.

Finally we must consider a variety of circumstances that have been said to precipitate schizophrenia. In considering these, it remains always essential not to confound the precipitant with the result of the illness.

SOMATIC FACTORS

Among the somatic factors childbirth is one of the more important ones. It is true that the first signs of a schizophrenic psychosis can appear after childbirth, and for schizophrenic women childbirth can bring about an exacerbation of the illness. However, many psychoses connected with childbirth are not of a schizophrenic nature and women who have had schizophrenic psychoses in the past do not necessarily relapse after childbirth. For the majority of the schizophrenic women childbirth does not influence the existing psychosis.

Occasionally a severe infectious illness can usher in a schizophrenic psychosis, but it also happens that schizophrenic patients experience a marked improvement, temporary or even permanent, during the course of a serious physical illness.

PSYCHOLOGICAL STRESS

Much has been written about environmental and other psychological stresses being responsible for the appearance of a schizophrenic psychosis. Some authors imply that such factors are the true cause of the illness, others think of them as precipitants. In their textbook, *Clinical Psychiatry,* Mayer-Gross, Slater, and Roth wrote: "It seems improbable that a severe mental illness leading to deterioration and destruction of the personality could be psychogenically determined, even if a strong genetic predisposition is assumed. One should, therefore, approach with skeptical reserve the rare cases in which a schizophrenic illness seems to be precipitated by emotional upset, mental conflict or other psychological or social difficulties." The author fully supports this viewpoint.

More often than not, one will find that the emotional stress a patient or his relatives claim to be responsible for the illness was itself the result of an insidiously beginning schizophrenic process. This is particularly true in cases where marital discord or difficult relations between a mother and her sick child are blamed for the appearance of the illness. It is easy to forget how difficult it is to live with a schizophrenic spouse or to bring up a schizophrenic child. Emotional diffidence, aloofness, and unpredictable behavior being the main characteristics of schizophrenia, one can readily imagine how they can lead to a tragic vicious circle in family relationships as long as the true nature of the behavioral changes is not recognized.

Furthermore, contrary to what one might expect, periods of great emotional stress, like the two world wars, confinement in concentration camps, or other major catastrophes, have not resulted in an increase in schizophrenic psychoses.

This is not to say that environmental stress or other psychological factors are never responsible for triggering the onset of a schizophrenic psychosis. Again, we like to think of such mechanisms in terms of our lock-and-key model, meaning that most probably a very specific traumatic incident is necessary to precipitate a schizophrenic psychosis in a person with a definite predisposition for this illness.

Finally, it must be recognized that in the same individual, schizophrenia can exist simultaneously with another mental disorder. Many schizophrenics drink or use drugs to excess. In these toxic phenomena, delirious conditions with specific hallucinations and delusions can mingle with schizophrenic ones. Schizophrenia can also be found in mental defectives, and the psychopathology will differ accordingly. Chronic brain syndromes due to arteriosclerosis or old age do not spare the schizophrenics and they, too, change the clinical picture, often by softening the schizophrenic symptoms. The symptoms of brain damage ultimately may completely obscure those of schizophrenia.

The Involutional Psychoses:

The concept of "involutional psychoses" is not well defined. In many textbooks the term is not mentioned and the psychoses under consideration are classified as belonging in part to the manic-depressive disorders and in part to the schizophrenias. This may well be correct. Obviously, age, personality, level of intelligence, and other factors modify these psychoses. Schizophrenia in a ten-year-old child presents a somewhat different clinical picture than it does in a person who takes ill at the age of forty, although in both cases it can be diagnosed as schizophrenia. From a psychological point of view it is easy to understand why, in an elderly person, a schizophrenic psychosis, or for that matter any mental illness, would acquire a paranoid or depressive flavor. Physiological involution takes place around the age of fifty in women and later in men. For many, particularly the mentally not so well balanced, dissatisfied persons, this period means the end of hopeful expectations and a reorientation in life, and depression would seem to be a natural reaction. Feelings of anger, disappointment, and self-depreciation are projected toward the environment and, in a paranoid fashion, sensed as ridicule and interference coming from others.

Definition: "Involutional" is the name for psychoses that appear during the years of physiological involution in persons who have not been mentally ill before. Their psychopathology is characterized by signs and symptoms of depression, of paranoid delusions, or by a blend of the two. Hallucinations without delirium are frequent; intellectual faculties are not affected.

DEPRESSIVE SYNDROMES

In all essential respects, the depressive syndromes are identical with those found in manic-depressive psychoses. Two features, however, often mark them as peculiar, namely, a general restlessness and agitation and the presence of rather absurd hypochondriacal delusions concerning various bodily functions. These patients, instead of quietly and dejectedly sitting in a corner, are apt to pace for hours, wringing their hands, lamenting loudly and clinging to nurses, doctors, and visitors. They will complain of the shriveling or the loss of their stomach, of an occlusion of the bowels, of a tumor or of the complete obstruction or the absence of all the vital "pipes" in the neck. Admittedly this symptomatology can be found in manic-depressive psychoses and can be absent in involutional psychoses. It may well be only a clinical "impression" that it is encountered more frequently in the involutional period.

Etiologically, the depression of late life, particularly when interspersed with paranoid delusions, remains as elusive as the other diseases described in this chapter. It is interesting to observe, however, that from a hereditary point of view it seems to belong to the group of schizophrenias rather than to the manic-depressive psychoses.

PARANOID SYNDROMES

The paranoid syndromes appearing for the first time during the involutional years differ little from the paranoid conditions described earlier, with the exception that auditory hallucinations and delusions concerning bodily functions are more prominent. Affectivity often appears slightly rigid but, in general, emotional contact remains good and thinking coherent. Thus these psychoses seem to assume a position in between paranoid schizophrenia and paranoid conditions.

Not infrequently, mild cerebral atrophy and symptoms of a beginning brain syndrome accompany the involutional psychoses. Some of the patients become easily confused and forgetful. In itself, however, the brain syndrome is not sufficiently pronounced to explain the psychosis. It may merely facilitate the precipitation of the psychosis by rendering the patient vulnerable to stress.

The courses of the involutional psychoses vary greatly. The depressive syndromes often clear up spontaneously within weeks or months, and they usually respond very well to somatic therapy. A few are difficult to treat, the psychosis taking a protracted course with only short-lasting temporary improvements.

The paranoid syndromes respond less well to treatment, and readily become chronic conditions, although there exist striking exceptions to this rule.

Some Statistical Information:

INCIDENCE

In the average population, the incidence of manic-depressive disease and schizophrenia is 0.4 per cent and 0.8-1.0 per cent, respectively.

AGE ON ADMISSION

A comparison of first-admission rates to hospitals according to age shows that the vast majority of schizophrenics are admitted between the ages of twenty and thirty, and that rather few are admitted after the age of fifty. For manic-depressive disease, the corresponding figures are thirty to fifty-five, and seventy.

LENGTH OF HOSPITALIZATION

Vera Norris has compared the average stay in mental hospitals of men aged thirty to thirty-nine years. She found that of the schizophrenic patients 16 per cent stay less than 10 weeks, 32 per cent stay between 10 and 29 weeks, and 44 per cent stay 52 weeks and longer. The corresponding figures for manic-depressive patients are 41.4 per cent, 36 per cent, and 15.8 per cent. It can be seen that schizophrenia appears early in life and that the chances of developing the illness are slim after the age of forty. On the other hand, the chances of leaving the hospital are good (50 per cent) only during the first two years. Thereafter, they decline rapidly.

Approximately half of all residents in public mental hospitals are schizophrenic patients, and the majority of them are between forty-five and fifty-four years old. These statistics do not show a breakdown according to subgroups, which would demonstrate significant differences among these subgroups.

Manic-depressive disease has its onset during a broader age range, the peak of which is displaced *to the right* by about thirty years in comparison to the one observed for schizophrenia. Over 75 per cent of the manic-depressive patients have left the hospital at the end of the 29th week, but there remain, nevertheless, 16 per cent who stay longer than 52 weeks. What might be concluded is that schizophrenia is not always as hopeless, and manic-depressive disease not always as benign an illness as one tends to believe.

Three Schizophrenic Patients:

Vera Sand, * born in 1916, was the daughter of a rather ordinary musician and a very bizarre mother. There were no known cases of mental disorder in the father's family. The mother, a religious fanatic, eccentric, restless, and litigious, was diagnosed as being schizophrenic. Two of the mother's four brothers committed suicide, one of them was hospitalized for schizophrenia. Her mother (Vera's grandmother) was hospitalized for schizophrenia and so were two of her twelve siblings. The two sisters and two brothers of Vera Sand had pronounced social difficulties because of egocentric and unproductive behavior.

Vera's childhood was erratic. She grew up in several different countries, went to many schools, learned four languages, and tried to mastermind her siblings at an early age. She was a difficult child, intelligent, overcritical, full of self-pity, and eccentric in her dressing and eating habits. Initially, she had many plans and expectations. She was active, studied business, switched to philosophy, and then to political sciences, but she did not finish anything.

At the age of twenty-five, she had spent great sums of money, had traveled restlessly, had no friends, had exhausted herself in bitter power struggles with her mother. A sudden state of excitement and vague paranoid ideas prompted a first hospitalization. Diagnosed as schizophrenic and treated with insulin, she was released from the hospital as improved after a stay of several months.

*All names are fictitious.

At this point, Vera had new but unrealistic plans. She thought of establishing a studio for rhythmic dancing, of another for photography, although she lacked the skill and talent for either. She wanted to set up a shop on wheels. Actually, she did nothing. She withdrew to a cabin at a lake. There she ruminated over the injustices committed by her mother, felt abandoned by all, and became more and more manneristic and unpredictable. At one period she ate enormously, at another, nothing; she wanted to be fat, then ethereal; practical, then intellectual. She walked around in pajamas, complaining that the room was too cold for her. Although she had with her twenty-three suitcases with clothes and other belongings, she wore the same dress every day. When she started to remain in bed, weighed no more than 80 pounds, was dirty and disheveled, her family once more interfered and took her to a mental hospital.

During many interviews and observations over a number of years, Vera consistently presented the same clinical picture. She was tall and slim, always wearing a tightly fitting black suit with a red belt, black stockings and shoes, no makeup. She moved slowly and although her movements appeared stiff, there was a catlike quality to them. Hardly ever was there an expression on Vera's face. Her muscles seemed to have no tone at all. During conversations she would open and close her mouth, saying astonishing things with wit and anger and intellectual acuity, but no twitching, no movement in her face, would verify or accentuate them. She would sit and talk monotonously and look out the window or stare at the wall. She remained distant, unconcerned, and timeless. Although her memory was perfect, her intelligence brilliant, and her judgment of those around her astute, the only matters she ever discussed were her mother, the resistance of the world, and the money and opportunities she had been denied. Of these things she spoke not always coherently, and what appeared logical and sequential to her was not to the listeners. She would contradict herself and lose her train of thought without noticing it. She would never accept anything others had to say to her. Although she claimed to be a perfect typist, she typed slowly and made many mistakes which she did not notice. She was never able to see her own performance and her behavior as others saw it. She was not hallucinated. Over a period of many years, she changed little. There was no shift in her almost nonexistent interests. She remained a quiet, autistic, and idle nonparticipating bystander in hospital activities, always adept in ducking, deviating, and obstructing plans designed to remotivate and mobilize her. Although she continued to protest blandly the legality of her confinement, she never tried to leave the hospital. All attempts to treat her with somatic and psychological means ended in failure.

Diagnosis: Simple schizophrenia.

Lucy Kent was born in 1928. She was brought to the hospital by her relatives. Her father, a simple man and laborer, made a peculiar impression. Whenever he looked at his sick daughter, he laughed strangely and inappropriately. The mother, intellectually dull, excited and insecure, forever talked about non-essential details with respect to the daughter's illness. Lucy's only sister, rigid and slow, appeared to be mentally ill. In 1942 she had had one "nervous breakdown," during which she was tired, apathetic, and mute. Since then, she had remained even more seclusive than she had been before the illness.

Lucy's birth and physical development were normal. As a child she was fearful, insecure, shy, and unduly dependent on others. She made no friends. She managed junior high school, became a seamstress, and did all her work in her parents' home. Her first psychotic episode lasted from February 1956 until April 1957. During this time she sat idle, ate almost nothing, reacted with hostility toward anyone trying to help her, and lashed out in abusive tirades against the torments of auditory, visual, and bodily hallucinations. She remained at home and without specific treatment recovered slowly. She did not resume her own work, but helped in the house.

New changes in her behavior were noticed on New Year's Day, 1959. She became rigid, apathetic, and negativistic. Although mildly depressed, she would suddenly burst out in unmotivated laughter, obviously in response to hallucinations. Again she remained at home without psychiatric treatment. In April 1960, she recovered and resumed her work as a seamstress, this time in a nearby town.

On April 26, 1962, she suddenly lapsed back into a deep catatonic stupor. Stiffly, she stood around, refused to eat or speak, and from time to time she produced a convulsive laughter or crying spell. This time she intimated suicidal ideas and therefore was taken to the hospital.

Until treatment was started, Lucy remained in bed, rigid, tense, and motionless. Food had to be given by gavage. Her facial expression never changed, but her eyes wandered around and observed carefully and correctly. At first, she remained mute, but then expressed ideas of guilt and delusions about having been a spy, or about being worthless and condemned. She heard voices which told her that she should not eat if she wanted to get better. Her physical health was good.

In May 1962, she was given electroshock treatment, and in June 1962, she was well enough to leave the hospital.

Diagnosis: Catatonic schizophrenia.

Encounter with a Paranoid Schizophrenic
While Making Ward Rounds:

"Good morning, Mr. Grant. How is it going?"

"All right, doctor. I had a visitor this morning."

"Oh, who was it?"

"Gloucester. You know, the Duke of Gloucester."

"Really? I wasn't told about it."

"It doesn't matter; we are going ahead!"

"Going ahead? How?"

"With plans. You have a new suit, correct? It looks OK."

"I am glad you like it, Mr. Grant."

"But I don't. I have made a petition. Haven't you seen it?"

"I have not, Mr. Grant. But you have been in this hospital for ten years and you must have sent me at least fifteen petitions requesting the re-evaluation of your trial. You know that the court has turned them all down. What do you want me to do now?"

"You just don't understand, doctor. The court means nothing. I have been here for nine years and six months, not ten years. You have to give the signal."

"Mr. Grant, I have told you many times that you should go into town and look for work, but you never do."

"That's not good enough. The plan asks for your signal—an unconditional release. Legally, I am the law. Do you understand? I sent you seventeen petitions not fifteen; you've got to be precise, doctor, with all that money waiting for me."

(Here we go again.) "If you have all this money coming to you, why don't you find a room and live on the outside, instead of folding sheets in the linen room."

"The President says no!"

"What do you mean, he says no? Did you hear him?"

"Certainly, he said it yesterday. He said it again just now."

"Voices, Mr. Grant?"

"Well, that's what you call them. But don't worry, you'll hear them when you need them. They will teach you. There is nothing wrong with folding linen."

"OK, Mr. Grant. I'm afraid that I'll have to be on my way now. I'll see you again tomorrow."

"Sure, doctor. Thanks for talking to me."

Mental Disorders of Known Etiology

(THE ACUTE AND CHRONIC BRAIN SYNDROME)

Introduction:

Presently, we will discuss the last group of mental disorders, which on our scale (page 49) are on the right end, indicating that from an etiological point of view, somatic factors are maximally demonstrable and essential, whereas psychological ones are of minor importance. In these disorders there exists a direct relationship between extent and location of the brain damage and the severity of the psychopathology. The brain damage may be diffuse, generalized, or circumscribed, and it may be anatomical or physiological in nature. The causes include hereditary genetic pathology, brain injuries, and metabolic, toxic, or degenerative processes. In American psychiatric nomenclature these disorders are called brain syndromes, and they are divided into two major groups: the acute and the chronic brain syndromes.

Acute brain syndromes are due to temporary, reversible brain damage. Many head injuries, acute intoxications with poisonous substances, and psychotic reactions accompanying infectious diseases are some of the prominent conditions of this category. The characteristic symptom is the clouding of consciousness.

Whenever irreversible, permanent, brain damage leads to psychopathology we speak of *chronic brain syndromes*. They can exist at birth or be acquired at any later stage of life. Severe forms of mental deficiency, brain damage due to chronic alcoholism, syphilis, and old age are well-known examples. The common denominator for these conditions is a personality change, in the sense of a personality deterioration with dementia of varying degrees.

Other symptoms found in brain syndromes concern disturbances in memory, thinking, and affectivity. In order to better understand this psychopathology, we shall take another look at the computer model described in the second chapter of this book.

Anatomical destruction or physiological malfunction, temporary or permanent, can befall any part of the brain. In computer terms, this would mean that all elements concerned with reception, translation, transmission, and output of information can be affected. Since the brain always functions as a physiological unit, as the computer does as an electronic one, disturbances in one area are likely to have repercussions in all others. However, inasmuch as certain anatomical and physiological structures of the brain are primarily concerned with specific functions, lesions in these areas will determine specific aspects of the psychopathology. For instance, lesions in the frontal parts of the brain are accompanied by changes in emotionality, and circumscribed irritations in the temporal areas may cause auditory hallucinations. In general the extent of the psychopathology will depend on the extent of the cerebral impairment. In this sense, the brain syndromes are unspecific, which means that many different illnesses will produce similar clinical psychopathology. There are exceptions to this rule and relatively minute destructions in certain key areas, in the midbrain for instance, can profoundly affect the entire physiology and mentality of the injured person, or put a very special stamp on an otherwise unspecific brain syndrome.

But let us return to the computer model. Alterations in the receiving elements will lead to basic distortions of information, to failures in registration and storage. Damage of elements concerned with the evaluation of information inhibits recall and proper availability of material for comparison and matching. Disturbance in the output system will produce faulty coordination and expression of information and commands. Translating this into medical language will help to understand the pathology in perception, intention, memory, and recall, in thinking, judgment, and verbalization. Accordingly, patients with brain syndromes often do not know where they are or who they are. They do not know the date or time, cannot remember happenings of the past, and are unable to recognize objects. Consequently, they cannot think properly. In order to cover up such deficits, patients make vague and general statements where precise ones are required, or liberally invent what they do not recall—a process called confabulation. Thus, asked in which town he lives, a patient may say "In a beautiful town," because he cannot recall the name of it. Another may explain that he had been working on his job all morning, although he has not had a job for years. Not being able to remember what he actually did this morning, he invents rather than acknowledge his incompetency.

More specific psychopathological symptoms will be discussed in connection with individual syndromes. Indeed, although the brain syndromes have basically the same structure, they vary greatly in intensity and details. Clinically, they may resemble neurotic, psychopathic, schizophrenic, or manic and depressive syndromes. However, the presence of a clouded consciousness, disorientation in time and place, memory deficits, or deterioration of intellectual faculties will reveal that this is only resemblance.

Often striking is the degree of reversibility of brain-syndrome symptomatology. A patient, today deeply beclouded, delusional, and hallucinated, may emerge from this condition tomorrow and look around in astonishment, not remembering anything of the automobile accident he had three days earlier.

Since the substrata of the brain syndrome are somatic afflictions of the brain, one must always expect to find neurological signs and symptoms together with psychopathological ones. This can be seen in injuries, infections, and tumors of the brain.

Since the symptomatologies are always similar, the author will describe only some of the most representative syndromes, rather than enumerate the many different afflications producing brain syndromes.

Acute Brain Syndromes:

Definition: Acute brain syndromes are psychoses due to reversible, diffuse anatomic or physiologic disturbances of the brain. In time they tend to appear and disappear together with the somatic dysfunction. The common symptom is a clouding of consciousness, but illusions, delusions, and hallucinations do occur. Sensations of extreme well-being or deep anxiety, of unreality and bodily distortion often arise. Irritability, overactivity, agitation, and elation, or apathy and depression mark the patient's behavior and mood. The acute brain syndromes accompany many different nonpsychiatric conditions.

1. *Acute Brain Syndromes in Infectious Diseases:*

At the height of a febrile illness, or sometimes preceding the rise in temperature, a patient may become somnolent or delirious. For minutes, hours or days, he may not know where he is, may misidentify nurse or doctor, misinterpret what is being said, and hear sounds nobody else can hear, such as the beating of drums, shooting, rattling, footsteps, or muffled voices. He may see faces appear and disappear on the walls, or see water around him and believe he is at a beach or in a swamp, and he may react accordingly by yelling, crying, and trying to get out of bed. Physical restraints or a strong sedative will be necessary to calm him down. As the patient overcomes the illness, the psychotic phenomena will fade and disappear.

Children are more prone to such psychotic reactions than are adults, but there exist great variations in susceptibility. It is not well understood what predisposes one person to become confused with each infectious disease he happens to catch, whereas another never seems to be so affected. The physiological processes involved are not clear. The fever as such does not seem to be responsible for the psychotic symptoms; more probably the toxic substances produced during the illness cause the reactions of the brain. Only in a few diseases, such as typhoid fever, have specific lesions been found in the brain.

Some of the most prominent diseases likely to be accompanied by an acute brain syndrome are rheumatism, influenza, typhoid fever, typhus, and malaria. In some cases, the damage done to the brain is not altogether reversible and lasting alterations in the personality or in intellectual faculties result. Typhus and rheumatism in children can have such consequences. Some authors believe that many psychopathic personalities suffered at an early age from such acute brain syndromes, which were not recognized, but left a lasting mark in the brain. If this were so, one would have to diagnose these cases as chronic brain syndromes and not as psychopathies.

With the advent of sulfanilamides and antibiotics, the natural course of most infectious diseases has been drastically altered, and acute brain syndromes in these afflictions are now less frequent. However psychiatrists are seldom consulted in such cases and statistics are not kept, so it is impossible even to guess the frequency of such syndromes. This is equally true in many of the illnesses to be discussed subsequently.

2. *Acute Brain Syndromes in Intoxication:*

During fall maneuvers in Germany, three American soldiers saw beautiful black berries hanging on a bush right next to their foxhole. Each took a handful and ate them. Within half an hour they felt strange, excited, and restless. Their vision became blurred and so did their minds. Confused and delusional, they left their duty station, and when other soldiers started to hold them, they became combative. Quickly taken to a nearby hospital, they were thought to be acutely schizophrenic and transferred to another hospital. Their widely dilated pupils, their great thirst and complaints of dry mouth, and finally their account of what had happened made it clear that they had eaten poisonous Belladonna berries. Within two days, they had recovered completely.

Belladonna is the basic substance of many useful drugs. There are other drugs which, taken in excessive quantities, produce toxic psychoses. The amphetamines (Dexedrine) prescribed for weight control, mood lifting, and taken as "boosters" by overworked students during examinations, are particularly dangerous because in addition to being habit forming, they produce acute brain syndromes in the form of a transient delirium, with disturbances of memory.

Barbiturates, morphine, cocaine, mescaline, and LSD25 are drugs or chemical substances that are usually taken intentionally, either for medical reasons or for "kicks," with the intention of bringing about a state of well-being, oblivion, or excitement. The last two mentioned are also being used to study "experimental psychoses." All of them produce acute brain syndromes.

It is believed that during rituals or in war, the ancient Norsemen used to eat certain mushrooms containing a chemical substance related to mescaline which would bring about heightened awareness, elation, ecstasy, fantastic hallucinations and delusions, and finally wild excitement. The term "going berserk" stems from this custom, a berserker being a Norseman frenzied in battle and believed to be invulnerable.

A final example of sad renown is the alcohol intoxication. The alcoholic admirably demonstrates all the phases encountered in acute toxic brain syndromes, from the initial feeling of well-being and friendly verbosity, through the stages of irritability, abusive language, and open hostility, to wild hallucinations, paranoid delusions, coma, and death.

Euphemistically, we distinguish between "normal" drunkenness, after which the person remembers what he did while intoxicated, and "pathological" drunkenness, after which the drinker has no recollection of what he has done. The day after a gay party at a friend's house, a middle-aged gentleman woke up in his own bed and found that he did not have the slightest idea of what had happened to him between about eight o'clock the night before and noon of the day he woke up. Frightened by this inexplicable interruption in his recollection, he ran to his garage where he found his car normally parked and without any dents or scratches. Not satisfied with this, he called the police station to find out whether or not there had been any accident during the night in which he could have been involved. There had been none. He called the friends at whose house he had been, and was told that he had been "just a little bit high, full of jokes and fun" and that he had driven away around midnight. Right then and there, this very reasonable gentleman stopped drinking. Pathological drunkenness is always indicative of a deeper mental disturbance.

After a number of years of steady and excessive drinking, the alcoholic may suddenly develop acute and dramatic delirious and hallucinatory states, lasting for days, weeks, or months. In these cases, vitamin deficiencies, together with the toxic effects of the alcohol, are responsible for the psychotic syndromes.

Best known of these psychoses is the delirium tremens, which often but not always starts at the moment of an interruption of the drinking pattern because of an accident or intercurrent disease. The increased needs of the body for defense and repair cannot be met and the psychosis begins. The patient becomes exceedingly tremulous, shaky, and restless. Soon he has visual hallucinations in the form of vivid scenes in which people and animals move and mill around, often playacting bits of his life history. He can hear these people talk to each other about him, his bad habits and his merits. He sees small animals crawling over his bed and up and down the walls. He may stumble around trying to catch them. For some, these events take on a rather funny character, but for many others, they are exceedingly frightening. Thus, one forty-year-old alcoholic man, in bed with delirium tremens, saw, heard, and felt a ferocious wolf under his bed who relentlessly snapped at his buttocks. In trying to get away, the patient kept jerking himself from one side of the bed to the other, despite heavy sedation, exhausting himself so completely that he died within a few days.

Delirium tremens is not a rare psychosis, and the mortality is still high, although much progress has been made in its treatment.

Obviously, acute brain syndromes can be the product of several noxious agents. Alcoholics often take drugs, particularly sleeping pills, and drug addicts experiment with many different compounds and frequently drink as well. Many people quite innocently take a variety of sedatives during the night, "pep pills" during the day, and here and there a couple of drinks until suddenly such a mixture proves to be too much for their body to tolerate.

The British novelist, Evelyn Waugh, has described such a condition in the delightful and most informative book, *Ordeal of Gilbert Pinfold*. Aldous Huxley tells about his experiences with the drug LSD25 in his book, *Doors of Perception*.

3. *Acute Brain Syndromes in Endocrine and Metabolic Diseases:*

Acute mental disturbances are being observed in affections of the adrenal and the thyroid glands. Patients with a hyperactive thyroid gland are over-alert, restless, and sleepless. This still benign condition can develop into an acute toxic psychosis, in many ways resembling a manic attack. Trembling hands, wide open shiny eyes, a clouded consciousness with memory disturbances, and other signs of hyperthyroidism will establish the correct diagnosis.

Severe renal diseases leading to an accumulation in the blood of toxic substances (uremia) are accompanied by clouding of consciousness and other psychotic phenomena.

Vitamin deficiencies, particularly those concerning the vitamin B complex, are apt to produce, at least initially, reversible brain syndromes. The most notable example is a disease called pellagra, found among poor peasants whose principal foodstuff is maize. The disease is frequently found in the countries surrounding the Mediterranean Sea, in the Far East, Africa, Mexico, and in the southern United States. Besides showing distinct neurological signs and a specific skin rash, the patients at first complain of fatigue and depression with suicidal ideas. Subsequently anxiety, irritability, and tension gradually progress to a delirious state with depressive overtones. Unless treated, the illness frequently ends in death.

Physical exhaustion and hunger can result in delirious, delusional, and hallucinatory states which disappear again as soon as the underlying physical condition has been corrected.

4. *Acute Brain Syndromes in Head Injuries and Brain Tumors:*

A head trauma can lead to a brain concussion, a condition in which there is temporary physiological interruption of function in parts of the brain. Concussions usually result from mild to moderate blows to the head, without skull fracture. In severe blows to the head, with skull fracture, and in stab or bullet wounds, the brain tissue is usually torn and hemorrhage occurs. This is called a contusion. There are exceptions to this rule, however, and sometimes an apparently very minor blow to the head results in a fracture of the skull, with or without contusion. Also, a mild trauma can rupture a blood vessel within the brain or on its surface without causing a fracture. As the amount of blood from the hemorrhage increases in size, pushing brain tissue aside or destroying it, the patient, who may have remained conscious after the blow, will become confused and unconscious. Almost all brain injuries are accompanied by more or less severe acute brain syndromes and many result in permanent damage and chronic brain syndromes. The location and extent of the injury determine the clinical picture to a certain extent. Again the common symptom is the clouded consciousness, ranging from a short-lasting daze to deep coma of several weeks' duration. During the period of clouded consciousness, the injured patient is usually restless, delusional, and often hallucinated. He does not realize where he is, misinterprets what is going on around him, and in this mood, vacillates between irritability and depression, hostile outbreaks and elation. He may eat normally and attend to his toilet needs, but he has much difficulty in retaining what he says, sees, and hears. Slowly, this confusion and restlessness will abate, and consciousness will clear up. However, the patient will probably remember neither the injury nor the events during the time of confusion. This period of amnesia or inability to remember may often cover a period of one or two hours preceding the injury. In this respect, it should be recalled what was said in Chapter II about fresh memory being constituted by reverberating electrical circuits involving a relatively small number of nerve cells. As we mentioned, mechanical interruption of these circuits will abolish fresh memory imprints in the same way that a blow at an electronic computer wipes out stored information.

Modern traffic, modern speed, and modern sports, particularly football and boxing, have made the traumatic head injury with acute brain syndrome a very frequent occurrence, but psychiatrists not affiliated with general hospitals may rarely see them.

Brain tumors impair brain function in two ways: 1) Located on the surface or inside the brain, they may push aside brain tissue as they grow in size. Since there is no room for expansion, the brain is compressed and pressure inside the skull rises. In the acute stage, particularly in fast growing tumors, this leads to an acute brain syndrome. Long-lasting compression of the brain causes brain atrophy and a chronic brain syndrome. 2) Brain tumors, particularly malignant ones, may destroy brain tissue at the site where they grow. In these cases, increased pressure may be minimal or absent, but the damage is permanent and a chronic brain syndrome will be the result, if the patient survives the removal of the tumor.

Chronic Brain Syndromes:

Definition: Chronic brain syndromes are abnormal mental conditions due to irreversible brain damage. The common symptom is a personality change and the most frequent additional syndrome concerns malfunctions in perception, recall, and memory.

Commentary: The abnormal mental condition can manifest itself in a permanent characterological or intellectual defect, such as post-encephalitic personality changes and mental deficiency, or in psychotic processes with delirium, delusions and hallucinations. Not infrequently we find a combination of the two conditions, as for example, when a mentally defective temporarily becomes psychotic.

The brain damage can be present at birth or acquired later; it can be hereditary or due to infections, metabolic diseases, toxic conditions, trauma, tumors, or old age. Almost all of the causes responsible for acute brain syndromes can produce chronic syndromes, provided their negative influence on the brain lasts long enough to bring about permanent damage. How crippling these syndromes will be depends on the extent and location of the lesion or lesions. The result of a brain injury can be no more than a character peculiarity or as much as a speechless, helpless, vegetating body nursed along for endless years.

Chronic brain syndromes are frequent, but the psychoses of old age constitute the majority of them.

1. *Chronic Brain Syndromes Associated with Infectious Diseases:*

Although many infectious diseases cause inflammatory lesions in the brain, and with them permanent damage, we will cite only two notable examples: epidemic encephalitis and syphilis.

Epidemic encephalitis, described and defined in 1917 by Constantin von Economo, a physician in Vienna, Austria, first appeared in 1915 in southeastern Europe. It remained epidemic for about ten years, spreading all over Europe and to some other parts of the world. Very few cases have been reported since.

It begins with an acute inflammation in the brain manifested by fever, headaches, general weakness, and malaise. The most characteristic symptoms are a disturbance in the sleep rhythm and mental changes. For days or weeks, the patients tend to sleep continuously, although they can be temporarily aroused for meals. Occasionally, the patients sleep only during the day, but remain awake during the night; a few cannot sleep at all.

This so-called lethargic state is accompanied or interrupted by delirious episodes with vivid and terrifying hallucinations, or by a stupor resembling the catatonic one described in the chapter on schizophrenia. Emotional reactions to external stimuli are peculiarly restricted and, at this stage, the patient's face seems to lose the ability to express feelings. Various neurological signs and symptoms are prominent, particularly with regard to eye movements.

Complete recovery occurred in about one fourth of the cases; in the remainder, the illness proceeded to a chronic stage lasting for many years and leading to permanent damage in distinct areas of the brain, particularly the so-called basic ganglia in the midbrain. The results are manifold, but characteristic in their composition of neurological and psychiatric symptomatology. The best known of the late syndromes is the post-encephalitic parkinsonism.

These patients hold themselves rigidly in a position bent slightly forward; their face is masklike and without expression, the mouth open and drooling. When they walk, they do so stiffly, with very small steps, and they look as if at the next step they will fall. Their fingers tremble, and they constantly make movements as if they were rolling pills between thumb and index finger. Their personality is markedly impoverished and their interests restricted. The patients are primarily concerned with themselves, although they have only limited insight for their condition and limitations. Intellectual faculties at first seem to be well preserved, but with the years there is a marked decline. Emotional lability is frequent and so are periods of depression. Many of these unhappy patients commit suicide.

If the acute illness strikes in childhood, the chronic course is different. These children become serious management problems. Although they retain their intelligence, they lose all control over their emotions. Overactive, over-alert, restless, mischievous, and distractible, they are troublesome at home and in public. Reasoning and punishment remain without effect and more often than not confinement in a mental hospital becomes unavoidable. In these cases, neurological symptoms are infrequent.

Since only a few cases of epidemic encephalitis have been reported since 1925, it is reasonable to expect that the post-encephalitic syndrome, as we still see it today, will become a clinical rarity.

Syphilis of the Brain: (A case of general paresis.)

George Lenz was twenty-five and in good mental health when he consulted a general practitioner for a rash on his body. Blood tests showed that he had syphilis of which the rash was a symptom. Treatment was begun, but Lenz found it bothersome and unimportant once the rash had disappeared. After a few sessions, he stopped going to the doctor. For the next fifteen years he worked as an accountant and did a creditable job. He married and led a quiet rather unremarkable life. His physical health seemed good. He had forgotten about the syphilis and never had his blood checked again.

When he reached the age of forty, those who worked with him noticed a change in his personality. At first it seemed that he became more friendly and outgoing, but soon this friendliness and jocosity proved to be rather shallow, trite, and silly, and not always in good taste. Progressively, Lenz lost his good manners and neglected his appearance. Into his previously conscientious work crept minor and subtle mistakes which soon were replaced by glaring ones. He would forget tasks he was told to do, although he would hold on to his daily routine. When questioned about the poor quality of his work, he did not seem to understand, and his superior found him peculiarly slow in his thinking. He was told to see a physician, but he took this advice lightly and quickly forgot it. Things got worse; he became more and more forgetful and dull. Finally, he was given a menial job in the warehouse, but there he could not orient himself at all. Within a week, he could no longer find his place of work, or recognize his new co-workers. In mid-January, he wore a summer suit and slippers. Over his loud and profane protestations, his wife took him to a physician, who in turn sent him to a mental hospital.

George Lenz was admitted to the hospital on January 24, 1936, at the age of 41, but he guessed that the date was August, 1922, and gave his age as 28 or 35. He greeted the admitting physician as his old friend and colleague, Peter, and told him that he had come to pay him a visit, mistaking the hospital for Peter's "nice new home."

Upon examination, his blood and spinal fluid both proved to be positive for syphilis. Showing obvious signs of a chronic brain syndrome in the form of a clouded consciousness, dementia, and personality disintegration, Lenz was diagnosed as having syphilis of the brain or, more precisely, general paresis. Penicillin did not exist at the time and the patient was treated with malaria fever, then the accepted form of therapy. This treatment was not successful, however, and during the following ten years, until his death, Lenz became more and more demented, apathetic, and neglectful in his personal hygiene. He never realized where he was, and formed various grandiose delusions regarding his own identity, which he quickly forgot and replaced with new ones. Occasionally he seemed to hear voices and sometimes at night he had visual hallucinations.

He died from pneumonia. On examination, the meninges or the sheets that envelop the brain were found to be of a milky discoloration and thickened. The brain itself was markedly shrunken and its gray matter, i.e., the part of the brain formed by the bodies of the nerve cells, was atrophic. Under the microscope few nerve cells were left, and many of them were distorted. The fine blood vessels were thickened from chronic inflammatory lesions, and a few spirochetes, the syphilitic agent, could be seen.

George Lenz represents a typical history of the chronic brain syndrome due to untreated or insufficiently treated syphilis. There are variations in the clinical picture, depending on which area of the brain and spinal column is attacked. The final result is always the same. Today, with syphilis under better control and the treatment of the late stages with penicillin more successful, this clinical picture is rapidly disappearing from our hospitals, a fact well reflected by statistics and the difficulties a teacher has in finding cases for demonstration to medical students and young psychiatrists.

2. *Chronic Brain Syndromes Associated with*
   Intoxication:

The brain has proportionally the largest oxygen consumption of any organ of the body. Lack of oxygen immediately produces functional and soon anatomical changes in the nerve cells. A number of poisons such as certain sleeping pills, anesthetics, carbon monoxide, and cyanide affect the oxygenation of the brain, and produce permanent damage in fairly specific areas.

Carbon monoxide, contained in illuminating gas, has an affinity to hemoglobin many times greater than that of oxygen, which hemoglobin is supposed to pick up in the lungs and carry to its destination. If carbon monoxide is present in the air, it combines with hemoglobin, replacing the oxygen and thus causing lack of oxygenation throughout the body but specifically in the brain. As a poison, it has an additionally damaging effect on the fine blood vessels of the brain. Illuminating gas has caused many accidents and it is a frequent means of committing suicide. About half of the persons who survive carbon monoxide intoxication remain permanently brain damaged. The resulting chronic brain syndrome is characterized by clouded consciousness, confusion, and memory defect. Headaches and parkinsonism, as described earlier, are frequently encountered.

Like chronic drug addiction, chronic' alcoholism can

lead to progressive destruction of brain tissue with severe personality changes, psychotic phenomena, and profound dementia. Every mental hospital has its share of these victims of an unfortunate habit.

3. *Chronic Brain Syndromes Associated with Old Age:*

Psychologically, we speak of aging when the past, the life we have lived, becomes so powerful that it over-shadows that part of life which we still have to live. (Ludwig Binswanger) Physiologically, aging is a process of progressive atrophy of all tissues and organs. In the brain, the number of nerve cells diminishes, the cortical gray layer becomes thin, and the convolutions narrow—the brain shrinks.

Aging is not a uniform process. Physiologically as well as psychologically some people show the first signs and symptoms of it at the age of sixty. Others, at ninety may have an atrophic skin and weak muscles, but their minds are as keen as they ever were. Although it may be generally true that most inventions have been made at an early age of the inventor, many a splendid book has been written and many a country admirably led by the very old. It is not fully understood what accounts for the differences in aging, but hereditary factors may well play an important role in it.

From a psychiatric point of view, the chronic brain syndrome due to aging differs little from other chronic brain syndromes except that its onset is late in life and that no cause other than old age can be elicited. The first symptoms are usually forgetfulness and a gradual loss of memory, particularly for recent events. The aged may well remember events of his childhood but not the headlines in the paper he just read. The grandmother may insist on making coffee but forget to put the coffee in the pot. In his mood the aged becomes labile, easily sheds tears, but laughs readily when consoled. Depressions are frequent but do not usually last long. Paranoid ideation is common and understandable. It seems natural for grandfather, who cannot find his glasses, to accuse the grandson of having put them away. Manners, dress, and personal hygiene are neglected. Control over emotional impulses may be seriously impaired, and since thinking becomes slow and befuddled and orientation in time and place defective, the aged gentleman may suddenly exhibit sexual misbehavior. He may urinate in public, reach under the waitress' skirt, or undress himself in front of little girls. The gradual loss of intellectual and ethical control often produces a caricature of the original personality. Thus the original spendthrift becomes a penny pincher, the devout a bigot, and the amusing storyteller a fantastic liar. However, as the dementia progresses these exaggerations lessen and a general dullness prevails, with occasional outbursts of temper. These patients increasingly need help when they dress and eat, when they search for the bathroom, or their beds. Throughout the illness, but more so during the advanced stages, delusions, hallucinations, and abundant irrational talk can dominate the clinical picture.

This chronic brain syndrome may begin at the age of seventy or eighty and develop slowly and steadily. If arteriosclerosis of the brain vessels is pronounced, the same syndrome may appear earlier and progress in a more erratic fashion, the deterioration being frequently interrupted by periods of a standstill or even improvement. The ultimate outcome is very much the same, but patients with cerebral arteriosclerosis are more prone than other old people to suffer cerebral hemorrhages and epileptic convulsions.

Two distinct chronic brain syndromes closely resemble the ones observed in old age. They have their onset at a much earlier stage in life and proceed swiftly, i.e., within a few years, to severe dementia and death. Often, they are called the presenile psychoses. The first one, *Alzheimer's disease,* shows pronounced cortical atrophy, particularly in the lateral parts of the brain and under the microscope presents an abundance of peculiar whorl-like patches of degeneration in the gray layers. Characteristically, these patients are constantly in motion, keeping up pseudo-activities. The etiology of this illness is not known.

In *Pick's disease* there is also marked cortical atrophy, but it is more circumscribed and restricted to the frontal and temporal lobes of the brain. Neurological signs such as speech impairments and epileptic seizures are prominent. This illness is hereditary.

4. *Chronic Brain Syndrome Associated with Brain Tumor:*

Jane Thorp was thirty-six years old when she voluntarily sought help in a psychiatric hospital. Her complaints centered around her marriage and her difficulties in controlling her temper in the never-ending disputes with her husband.

As a child Jane had been somewhat oversensitive, but she did well in school, was sociable, interested in sports and music, and prior to her marriage she worked successfully as a secretary. She met her husband when she was twenty-five and they were married soon after. He was her senior by ten years, quite independent, unromantic, but loyal and sympathetic toward her and their two children. Until about one year prior to admission to the hospital, the marriage seemed free of serious friction. At that time, Jane increasingly resented what she felt was her husband's aloofness and in long discussions she openly expressed these feelings. He promised to change, but as time went on she became more unreasonable in her demands and he more irritated about her. Crying spells, outbursts of anger, slamming of doors, sleepless nights, and nights with nightmares followed. The daily discussions started to center around divorce, and finally Jane moved out of the house. Her family physician, whom she consulted for her irritability and sleeplessness, advised that both she and her husband visit a psychiatrist to straighten out their problems. The husband refused, but the patient decided to come to the hospital.

On admission she felt well physically, but was tired, mildly depressed, and disgusted with life. She was perfectly rational, emotional contact with her was good, and she told her story in a coherent, somewhat exaggerated, but nevertheless convincing way. Psychological tests corroborated the initial clinical impression of a psychoneurosis. There was no evidence of any organic brain damage. Physical examination revealed no pathology, except that the right eyeground showed mild swelling in the center, a sign that could indicate increased pressure within the skull.

With this latter fact in mind, Jane was asked about headaches. She had never had any. However, the next day she complained of frontal headaches. She was asked about blurred vision. She had never had any, but the following morning she reported blurred vision. To the young psychiatrists this confirmed their suspicion that the patient was a neurotic woman with marked hysterical suggestibility, in dire need of immediate psychotherapy. However, the medical director shook his head and ordered an examination of the spinal fluid; since the first skull X ray had not shown anything of significance, he had additional films taken. Unfortunately for the patient and as an everlasting lesson to the young psychiatrists, the medical director found what he was looking for—an already large, slow-growing tumor in the frontal lobe of the brain. It could be removed only partially and six months later Jane died.

This, too, is the story of a chronic brain syndrome. It shows that a tumor or any other insidious brain damage in the frontal lobe can bring out dormant emotional conflicts which for a long time may overshadow all other symptoms of a slow compression of the brain. It shows that the personality change can precede all changes in perception, recall, and memory, and it finally demonstrates the importance of a thorough training in neurology for the psychiatrist and the necessity of establishing a well-founded diagnosis prior to embarking on therapy.

5. *The Chronic Brain Syndrome Associated with Idiopathic Epilepsy:*

The outstanding symptom of epilepsy is the seizure or convulsion. It consists of a sudden loss of consciousness with suspension of breathing, a period of general muscular rigidity, followed by rhythmic spastic movements of all extremities. With the last convulsive movement, breathing sets in, and the epileptic regains consciousness. The entire seizure lasts one or two minutes. During the seizure the recordings of the brain waves show characteristic electric discharges that are different from the equally specific discharge patterns found in between seizures. There are a number of variations in the types and frequencies of epileptic seizures.

In the most general terms, the epileptic seizure is the result of sudden abnormal electric discharges of nerve cells within the brain, due to circumscribed irritations or lesions. As such, seizures can occur as one symptom among others in a variety of diseases of the brain. High fever in an infectious illness with cerebral involvement, acute toxic conditions, brain tumors, cerebral atrophy in old age, and cerebral arteriosclerosis are some of the conditions that are possibly but not necessarily accompanied by symptomatic convulsions.

In the majority of epileptics, however, no such causation is known, and in these cases we speak of idiopathic or genuine epilepsy. Idiopathic epilepsy has been a bone of contention between neurologists and psychiatrists. In Europe it is dealt with in the textbooks of psychiatry, in the United States in those of neurology. For decades the European psychiatrists have stressed the psychiatric, and the American authors the neurological, aspects of the disease. That epilepsy is a disease entity has been doubted and some workers are confident that all epilepsies will ultimately turn out to be symptomatic in nature. Undoubtedly, successful modern treatment of seizures has done much to change the clinical picture as we so frequently saw it during the first quarter of this century. But the equally new and modern knowledge from brain wave tests and psychological tests tends to revive interest in some of the earlier findings and "clinical impressions."

The psychiatrist is concerned with three aspects of epilepsy. First, a certain number of epileptics develop all the characteristic signs and symptoms of a chronic brain syndrome, particularly a personality deterioration and dementia. Among these are primarily the ones who cannot be treated successfully and continue to have convulsions over a long period of years.

The psychiatrist is also concerned with the fears and phobias the epileptic acquires with respect to his own illness. The expectation of another seizure, perhaps in a busy street, at work, or at a party, can have crippling effects on the emotional and social life of the epileptic. In this he may need psychotherapeutic help in addition to anticonvulsive medication. It is a peculiar fact, however, that many epileptics remain overly confident and unconcerned, forever believing that their most recent seizure was their last. This often creates difficulties in therapy, inasmuch as the patients refuse to continue to take their medication once the convulsions are under control. They do not realize that our present treatment is only symptomatic and not curative.

The third point of interest and concern is the so-called epileptoid character. The old experienced clinicians knew it well as something to reckon with. One encounters this character type in many epileptics with seizures but also in persons with certain personality disorders without seizures.

Brain wave tests in the latter show a surprisingly high incidence of brain wave patterns suggestive of epilepsy.

Instability and simultaneous dominance of mood are most significant of the epileptoid personality. Moods change quickly at the slightest provocation and entirely dominate thinking and behavior. Thus anger can be extreme and vicious and result in sudden unexpected criminal acts; love may be so sweet as to be intolerable. These moods are tenacious and take their course, so to speak, until they are replaced by others, equally extreme and vicious. A person with such a character structure is difficult to deal with and one must always be on guard lest one offend him.

For more detailed description of idiopathic epilepsy, the reader is referred to the textbooks on neurology.

Mental Deficiency (Idiopathic):

Mental deficiency can be a symptom of a chronic brain syndrome or an independent illness. If the brain is injured during its formative period, be this before birth or during the very first years of life, a chronic brain syndrome results, of which mental deficiency can be a symptom. Clinically, the symptomatology and the medical and social problems encountered are the same in symptomatic and in idiopathic mental deficiency.

The original concept of mental deficiency as a unitary disease could not be maintained as new and very different etiologies were discovered. However, there still remain a number of cases in which the etiology is not known and others which are clearly of a hereditary nature.

It must be understood that in this chapter we will not deal with those mild cases of deficiencies which merely constitute variations within the normal range of intelligence, but only with mental deficiency as an illness.

Definition: Mental deficiency or retardation is characterized by a permanent defect in intelligence and personality, usually present at birth or apparent shortly thereafter, due to arrest or retardation of the normal intra- or initial extra-uterine development of the brain. The etiology is not uniform and to a large extent is still unknown. In the majority of cases, the degree of deficiency cannot be influenced by therapy.

The level of intelligence is the central issue in mental deficiency. There are many definitions of intelligence, each having merits and shortcomings. Louis William Stern's definition appears to be appropriate for our purpose: "Intelligence is the general ability to adapt to new situations by means of purposeful thinking." Intelligence comprises a variety of individual faculties, such as apperception, the ability to retain, to recall, and to remember what has been seen, heard, felt, or thought. It also includes the ability to pay attention and to express thoughts in speech and motor actions. Characteristic of the defective are his inability to judge, his intellectual shortsightedness, his inability to understand the larger context, the abstract meaning of a problem, and in general, his lack of interest.

However, mere defect in intelligence never encompasses the mental defective as we encounter him. The intellectual deficit is always embedded in an impoverished and restricted personality.

Classification:

Intelligence can be assessed quite accurately by psychological tests. These tests express the level of intelligence by means of an intelligence quotient (I.Q.). According to such tests an I.Q. between 90 and 110 represents average intelligence, I.Q. above 110 indicates "bright normal" and "superior," and I.Q. of 81 to 89 indicates "dull normal" intelligence.

Mental deficiency has been classified into three categories according to I.Q. levels:

1. Mild mental deficiency with I.Q. of 71 to 80. Children with such I.Q.'s can follow in school if placed in special classes. In later life they can earn a marginal subsistence by doing simple menial jobs.

2. Moderate mental deficiency with I.Q. of 51 to 70. Children in this I.Q. range cannot be taught in regular schools but need special, mostly institutional training and guidance. As adults, most of them are not able to support themselves.

3. Severe mental deficiency with I.Q. below 50. This group includes the imbeciles and idiots. Complete custodial and protective care is needed in most of these cases. Many of them can neither speak, dress, nor feed themselves.

Symptomatology:

To the observant mother a serious degree of retardation in her child becomes evident during the very first months of life. Every phase of a normal development is delayed—for instance, body movements, following objects with the eyes, turning, sitting up, standing, speech, and toilet training.

Mental deficiency is not an isolated phenomenon in an otherwise normal person. It is all-pervasive and can be noticed in the defective's facial expression, his gait and other movements, in his speech, his emotional responses, his reasonings, and in his motivations. A term embracing all this would be "lack of differentiation." Movements, including speech, are clumsy because of poorly differentiated coordination; affective reactions lack the fine shadings we are accustomed to gauge in normals; thinking is concrete and motivations crude because of the poverty of reflections and available memories.

The defective's abilities to perceive accurately and to put together, to compare, evaluate, and judge what he has perceived are impaired. He does not learn. He lives forever in the present because he can neither think in abstract terms nor plan for the future. A defective can learn to buy one loaf of bread for twenty-five cents, but when asked the price of two loaves of bread, he may answer "I don't know, I never buy two." He may be able to tell the number of apples there are if told that Ann, Peter and Jane each have three. But if he were asked how much is three times three, he could not answer. Many mental defectives are pleasant, friendly, and easy to guide. Others are stubborn, erratic, and unpredictable. Dysphoric moods, sudden outbursts of anger and hostility are frequent and easily triggered by minor incidents in which the defective does not get his way. Because of their gross lack of good judgment and foresight, defectives may at such moments commit serious crimes, including murder. One Saturday a farmhand fed a horse a handful of nails. The horse had to be killed and the nails were found in its stomach. The farmhand explained that he wanted to take off on Sunday afternoon, but he knew that he could not do this if he had to feed the horse. It seemed natural to him to do away with the horse. He had an I.Q. of 52; charges against him were dropped.

Frequently, mentally defective women are sexually promiscuous and become prostitutes. Alcoholism is another problem which often befalls the defectives.

How much the defective can learn and how well he will do in life depends on the level of his intelligence, but also on the amount of care, training, parental love, and moral support he receives. Being dependent on others makes the defective particularly vulnerable to ridicule, coldness, and rudeness. Parents have to bear this in mind when they set goals for such a child. To be kept in a class which requires more skill than the child has can be more traumatic than helpful. Classmates usually are cruel to the defective, and unfortunately many a teacher lacks in understanding; thus, every school day may represent an ordeal and a tragedy for the defective child who could possibly learn quite well and happily in a class for defective children.

The lower the intelligence level the more frequently we find physical abnormalities, such as deformities of the skull, or malformations of the spine, the extremities, or inner organs.

Etiological Considerations:

Many etiological factors have to be considered. There are undoubtedly families with hereditary mental deficiency and some countries have sterilization laws for such cases. In other instances, gene mutations have to be considered, as well as toxic influences on the germ plasm of one of the parents. Infectious diseases of the mother during pregnancy, particularly German measles, may have adverse effects on the nervous system of the fetus. Brain injuries sustained during prolonged or otherwise difficult deliveries and diseases of the newborn may also be responsible for mental deficiency. The assumption that an unfavorable environment can cause mental deficiency has to be viewed with great caution and skepticism. Mental deficiency hardly ever leads to prosperity, and rarely is a defective parent an ideal educator. It may be impossible in such cases to disentangle the etiological responsibilities.

There are special forms of mental deficiency with well-established etiologies. Cretinism is due to a non-functioning thyroid gland. Cretins do not grow to normal size, show various physical abnormalities, and very marked mental deficiency. Mongolism is due to a chromosomal abnormality, the genesis of which is obscure. These children remain small, are usually severely defective, but good tempered. They rarely reach the age of fifteen. Phenylketonuria is a newly discovered type of mental deficiency. In these cases a metabolic defect, i.e., the lack of a specific enzyme necessary to metabolize phenylalanine, causes the mental deficiency. If a diet low in phenylalanine is fed to these children their condition improves. Urine tests aid the diagnosis of the illness. The disorder is transmitted genetically by a single recessive gene.

Anatomical findings in the brain vary greatly with the etiology and degree of the mental deficiency. In mild cases the brain may be perfectly normal in appearance and microscopic examination of its tissues remains unrewarding. In severe mental deficiency, the brain may be very small, with narrow convolutions and a very thin cortical layer. In addition, there can be enlargement of the cavities within the brain, known as internal hydrocephalus. Many other abnormalities, diffuse, unilateral, or bilateral, can exist.

Incidence. It has been estimated that there are about 2,400,000 mental defectives in the United States of America. Other figures give a much higher incidence of 5 per cent of the general population. Over 200,000 mental defectives reside in special institutions. By far the greatest percentage of the total number of mental defectives have I.Q.'s above 50, but of those hospitalized the majority are suffering from severe mental deficiency. Although petty criminality occurs relatively frequently among the retarded, the percentage of recognized mental defectives among prison populations is allegedly less than one per cent. However, some authors have estimated that at least 10 per cent of all criminals are mentally retarded.

E. O. Lewis in England tested representative samples of all school children in various parts of England and ascertained by all available means the adult mental defectives in the same areas. In a total population of over 600,000, he found over 5,000 defectives of whom 5 per cent were idiots, 20 per cent imbeciles, and 75 per cent feeble-minded. The total incidence of 8 per 1,000 must be regarded as a minimum for England and Wales. However, other studies indicate a much higher incidence of mental deficiency in the general population.*

*Mayer-Gross, Slater, and Roth, *Clinical Psychiatry,* p. 61.

·VII·

Management

*"Whenever we accuse and judge
we miss the essential."*
   P. VALERY.

General Remarks:

This chapter is concerned with the treatment of the mentally ill. The term "management" has been chosen because in psychiatry therapy transcends the prescribing of medication and other strictly medical procedures. Invariably it includes social rehabilitation or reorientation of the patient and his environment. Physicians, nurses, and occupational therapists, social workers, teachers, members of the family, and sometimes judges, are all involved in a comprehensive therapeutic program that may start before the patient enters a hospital and end a long time after he has left it. We call this program management.

The reader may ask why the author has chosen to assign a special chapter to management instead of adding to each section a paragraph on therapy dealing with individual diseases. As mentioned initially, the author is concerned with discussing basic issues and problems in the hope of conveying a general understanding of psychiatry.

In adding remarks on treatment to each section, frequent repetitions and cumbersome explanations could not have been avoided. At times a variety of diseases may require the same kind of therapy, whereas a single disease may, at different times, need different therapeutic approaches. These and other reasons made it seem preferable to discuss principles of management rather than treatment of individual cases.

Possibilities and limitations in psychiatric management deserve some introductory remarks. Almost every mental patient who comes to seek help has potentialities for improvement, but there are intrinsic limitations as to how far this improvement can progress. For the therapist, it is imperative to know about both. The mental defective trying to compete with normal children in the hope of pleasing his parents is miserable and stands in his own way. Advice to the parents, guidance for the child, and changes in the scholastic program can provide satisfaction and happiness to both parents and child. The child's limitation is his mental deficiency, which no medication and no fine program can alter. It is cruel and unjustified to abandon the confused, depressed, and unhappy senile grandmother because "after all she is eighty-two years old and nothing can be done anyway." Actually, there is much that can be done for her. Electroshock therapy, for instance, can lift her depression and render her quite content. Her limitations are the senile atrophy of the brain, and while shock therapy will not increase her memory deficit and her confusion, it will lessen the depression. If left alone some schizophrenics would sit for years in the same corner of a room. An active ward program can prevent this kind of deterioration. The patient's limitations are intrinsic in the malignant type of schizophrenia which has frustrated all other therapeutic attempts.

Over the past one hundred and fifty years the pendulum has swung back and forth between therapeutic enthusiasm and resignation. Not counting modern somatic therapies, there is hardly anything we do today which was not done in the past in one form or another. Presently, it is being rediscovered that of the 600,000 patients in our mental hospitals many could very well live gainfully outside. "Push programs" are being designed and efforts are being made to treat new patients without admitting them to mental hospitals. This is all very well. The possibilities for successful treatment are great and many had been neglected in the past. However, here, too, are limitations. A patient who has been "pushed out" of the hospital and lives with his family is not necessarily well or even improved just because he is at home. He may be as ill as he was before, and in addition, unhappy and disrupting the family life. The only one satisfied is an overzealous doctor out to prove a point or to "improve" his statistics. Realism is better than either unwarranted enthusiasm or pessimism. It is a reality that all branches of medicine have their successes and their failures.

What we may call a therapeutic success and what a failure is depends on the goal we set in each individual case. If the goal is a realistic one, success can be expected. The psychotherapist who sets out to make over his psychopathic patient is apt to become disenchanted. If his goal is to help the patient to better control some of his impulses, he might be successful. To promise a mother that her hebephrenic daughter will be cured within a few months is irresponsible. It would be more realistic to express hope that after initiation of drug therapy the girl may well need less supervision and be able to return home.

There is nothing despicable about setting limited goals. After a bad crash a Cadillac can be repaired, but nobody will be surprised that its value has suffered. If a boy has a cancerous growth on his knee, the surgeon amputates his leg, but if the boy has diabetes he will have to take insulin for the rest of his life. These are all unpleasant realities met successfully by the setting of limited goals. Thus, unless we have the means to cure, the therapeutic goal in medicine is compensation of function. In this the psychiatrist does quite well.

Since little is known about the etiologies of the major psychoses, our therapeutic goals must center primarily around relief of symptoms and compensation of functions. The new psychoeffective drugs have brought about particularly decisive changes in this respect. Today, patients who once were kept on locked wards go home on weekends; others never reach the hospital because they can be treated in the physician's office. On continuous medication, a schizophrenic clerk may work and be fairly happy although he still hears a few voices and cannot entirely suppress his suspicions. If this is all treatment can do for him at this time, the clerk is still as successfully compensated as is the person who takes digitalis to keep in check his failing heart.

In order to evaluate successes and failures and to do justice to the doctors' skill we must know something about the natural course of mental diseases. It has been said that half of the neuroses remit spontaneously and it is well known that almost all depressions lift after they run their course. The physician who is being called on the scene just at the right moment is lucky. Many a "miraculous cure" has been effected in schizophrenics. Unfortunately, the "good" treatment usually fails in other patients who do not happen to be in spontaneous remissions at the time of treatment. The therapist must retain an honest and critical attitude toward his own therapeutic activities. He may deserve less praise when he succeeds, but he also deserves less blame when he fails.

TREATMENT PLAN

Management should proceed along a well-considered treatment plan. The different steps must begin with the establishment of a diagnosis and the evaluation of the patient's potentialities for cure or improvement and his probable limitations in this respect. This includes an appraisal of his home situation. Next, the therapeutic goal can be set and the means chosen by which it is hoped to reach it. At this point, the treatment begins, progress is reviewed at regular intervals to permit adjustments whenever necessary.

A limit in time ought to be set for the treatment plan. The author has never ceased to be amazed by the generosity with which psychiatrists dispose of their patients' time. In a mental hospital the smallest time unit known does not seem to be a minute or an hour but the week. Often a time limit has a stimulating effect on the patient, his relatives, and the doctor as well. The character of mental diseases changes with time. Some, like manic-depressive psychoses, are cyclic in nature, each depression or elation being limited in time. Under treatment, however, these natural time boundaries may become unrecognizable. This is important to know. If, for instance, drug treatment is discontinued too early, the depression may reappear. Schizophrenia is usually a phasic illness, i.e., periods of relative quiescence alternate with periods of exacerbation of symptomatology.

It is at present a question of controversy whether or not certain schizophrenic patients ought to be kept on drug treatment indefinitely. Experiences with large-scale discontinuations of drug therapy on hospital ward populations show that many patients do not need the medication they receive. This does not mean that they did not need it when it was first prescribed, nor does it imply that they will not need it again in the future. However, taking into account the phasic nature of the illness, one must at regular intervals find out whether or not drugs are still needed. This is all the more important since psycho-effective drugs are not harmless and should not be given if they are not needed. The therapist does well to always have in mind the cyclic, phasic, or continuous pattern of a given psychopathology.

What is being treated?

In acute brain syndromes we often treat the causes of the syndromes, inasmuch as we try to eliminate them as quickly as possible. One removes the victim from the room in which he has tried to asphyxiate himself with illuminating gas, and does everything possible to re-establish normal oxygen supply to the brain. In chronic brain syndromes we treat the alcoholic by withholding alcohol and the paretic by destroying the syphilitic spirochete with penicillin. And, theoretically at least, psychotherapy attempts to eliminate the cause of the neurosis.

However, the majority of the serious psychiatric casualties suffer from schizophrenia, manic-depressive disease and psychoses due to old age. In these as in other less frequent mental diseases, the therapy is a symptomatic one, that is, we treat symptoms or syndromes since we either do not know the causes or are unable to eradicate them. The physician who treats a diabetic patient with insulin does the same thing. He corrects the symptom, the abnormal sugar level in the blood, but leaves unaltered the original pathology in the pancreas. His patient continues to have diabetes, even though he is symptom-free as long as he takes his medication. Similarly, what we called the compensated schizophrenic remains a schizophrenic although his most bothersome symptoms may be controlled by drugs.

Most of the therapeutic tools we possess are not disease specific. There is, for example, no therapy that would be used exclusively in schizophrenia, in one schizophrenic subtype, or in depressions. Electroshock therapy, drug therapy or psychotherapy find their application in a wide variety of diseases. A psychotic depression or a catatonic stupor can be treated by drugs or with electroshock therapy. Under such circumstances, the specificity of our therapeutic agents is symptom- or syndrome-directed. Thus there are drugs that are specific mood lifters, others that are primarily tranquilizers or sedatives. Some drugs combine activating, antidepressive, and sedative effects. Electroshock has a specific antidepressive effect, but can also be used in breaking through manic excitement and catatonic stupor.

Thus, the initial choice of a specific therapy is based on a critical evaluation of what have been termed target symptoms (Freyhan), i.e., of the outstanding symptoms and their responsiveness to one or the other therapeutic agent. If target symptoms are known to respond to several therapeutic methods, for instance to drugs as well as to electroshock, the choice between these may be dictated by individual preferences of physician or patient, or by the availability of time and hospital facilities.

A final comment must be made about the important fact that the physician never treats an illness but always a sick individual. At least to a certain extent, almost any illness is being transformed by the character and the physical and moral strength of the person who suffers from it. Of two patients with ankle fractures, one may have to be told to take it easy and the other not to sit all the time. In mapping out the overall management, it is important to know the patient's attitude toward his illness and how he deals with it. Similarly, we have to take into account the attitude the relatives assume toward the patient. Thus, we have to consider the primary symptoms of the illness itself, and the secondary symptoms and problems created by attitudes concerned with the illness and the mentally ill. It is often difficult to determine which set of problems is the most harmful.

Obviously then, etiological or symptomatic, treatment always focuses on several aspects, different in nature and, as time passes, shifting in importance. The treatment of an acutely depressed mother of three small children is focused on a very specific problem of great urgency. Therapy for an acutely schizophrenic young man rests on premises, hopes and assumptions not applicable in the treatment of a chronic schizophrenic who has been in and out of mental hospitals for a period of twenty years.

At this point, we should conclude these general remarks with a discussion as to where treatment is to be undertaken and by whom. The author will elaborate on this topic under the heading "Outlook" at the end of this chapter. In the following pages the reader will find a brief account on some of the modern treatment modalities, their indications and limitations, and finally a short review of special management problems in some of the most important mental diseases.

SOMATIC THERAPIES

Psychoeffective Drugs:

In one form or another drugs have always been used in the treatment of the mentally ill. During the first half of this century barbiturates, bromides, and opiates were given to agitated, fearful, tense, and depressed patients. The results were usually short-lived and unsatisfactory.

In the early fifties new drugs were discovered which proved to be more specific in suppressing and changing psychiatric symptoms. From France came the first (chlorpromazine) of the now well-known tranquilizers. In the United States and elsewhere psychiatrists took notice of reports from internists stating that the drug isoniazid, used in the treatment of tuberculosis, had mood-lifting qualities. Since then, many other chemical compounds with antidepressive actions have been found and used.

Chemically, the most important tranquilizing drugs are phenothiazines. All of them have this nucleus:

(Fig. 3)

Modifications in the sidechains at positions R and R^1 determine the differences among the many commercially available phenothiazines.

Sedation:

Pharmacologically, these drugs have specific effects on circumscribed areas of the central nervous system. Clinically, their most desirable action is the inducement of sedation without reduction in awareness. They promote sleep from which the patient can be aroused easily. Some clinicians believe that the tranquilizers have a direct inhibitory action on delusions and hallucinations, others tend to think that the disappearance or diminution of hallucinations and delusions is a secondary phenomenon due to the primary reduction of inner tension and anxiety.

At normal dosage levels and more so at high dosage levels, the phenothiazines and the less frequently used Rauwolfia derivatives have very marked effects on the neuromuscular system. Muscular tension is increased, movements become slow, infrequent, and smaller in amplitude. A fine tremor will be noticeable in the fingers and hands and frequently the patient will experience a peculiar restlessness, manifested by continuous shuffling of the feet, and an inability to sit still or to stay in one place. The reader will have noticed that in many ways these tranquilizers produce a clinical picture not unlike the one we saw in the late stages of epidemic encephalitis. This fact represents intriguing theoretical and practical problems. For instance, the question has arisen as to whether or not one ought to consider these neurological signs and symptoms to be undesirable side effects of the drugs. Most clinicians, however, hold that the symptoms are essential and it has been shown that phenothiazines which do not produce them are therapeutically ineffective. These symptoms are reversible, that is, they disappear with the reduction in dosage or the discontinuation of the drug. If they become too bothersome, it is possible to attenuate them with other drugs. (See page 130.)

The phenothiazines differ from one another primarily in potency. Some of them have depressive, and others slightly mood-lifting and psychoactivating, properties. In general, there is little justification in shifting therapy from one of these drugs to another of the same type, and it is safe to say that if one or two phenothiazines are totally ineffective in a particular case, others will not be of much help either.

Therapeutic Indications of Tranquilizers:

Target symptoms of the first order are all states of physical and emotional excitement and restlessness. Such conditions, as seen in manic attacks, or in acute or chronic brain syndromes, respond within half an hour to an adequate dosage of a potent phenothiazine. Further, states of inner tension and anxiety, expressed in stiff, rigid, and frozen attitudes often combined with paranoid ideations, respond well to these drugs. Here, for instance, we think of the tense, catatonic, and mute patient who refuses to eat and the paranoid who believes himself caught in the nets of his persecutors, or of the person with a severe anxiety neurosis. Usually, chronic conditions with marked motor overactivity, such as hebephrenia, and some senile and other brain syndromes respond favorably to medium doses of tranquilizers.

Hallucinations and delusions, in the author's opinion, are not target symptoms for drug therapy. However, they often do disappear with the tranquilization of the patient's anxiety and tension. But, equally, an excited and tense paranoid patient with many delusions and hallucinations may become quiet and relaxed under the influence of drugs, but still retain his delusional ideas and continue to hear voices. Tranquilizers are not indicated in depressions, since they will only deepen the depression and possibly precipitate suicide. Only in agitated depressions can it be an advantage to combine a mild tranquilizer with an antidepressive drug.

DANGERS AND SIDE EFFECTS

Obviously, tranquilizers are being prescribed in a host of other conditions—in the author's opinion, altogether too frequently. In many cases of nervousness, sleeplessness, and mild anxieties some of the older sedatives would be more appropriate. It must never be overlooked that the phenothiazines and other tranquilizers are not at all harmless drugs. They cause immediate and long-range side effects, many of them due to the atropine-like effects of these drugs. Some most frequently encountered side effects are: tremor of the hands, dryness in the mouth, dizziness, constipation, and more rarely general muscular stiffness, blurred vision and sudden drop in blood pressure upon changing of position of the body. More serious are liver damage and changes in blood morphology. In patients who take large amounts of these drugs over a period of several years we may occasionally find opacities in the cornea and lens of the eyes, and rarely permanent neurological symptoms marked by involuntary movements of muscles of the face, neck, arms and legs. Death due to liver, blood and heart damage has been reported. However, it must be emphasized that almost all of these symptoms are reversible and quickly disappear when the dosage of the drug is being reduced. All these drugs should only be taken under the constant supervision of a physician who uses due precaution to avoid unhappy complications.

Since the first edition of this book in 1964 a number of new psychoactive drugs have become available. Many of them are variations of the original phenothiazine (Thorazine), and of another originally French tranquilizer Haloperidol. So far none of them have resulted in striking improvements in psychopharmacology. Of some interest are oily solutions of a potent phenothiazine that can be given intramuscularly. They are absorbed very slowly over a period of ten to 30 days, and thus eliminate the need of daily administration. The advantage of such drugs is that we can be sure that the patients are really being kept on the drug; their disadvantage is that once administered, the physician has lost his freedom to reduce the dosage for 2 weeks following the injections. Obviously, one has to be thoroughly acquainted with the patient's course of illness and his way of reacting to the same drug in its original form.

A probably far reaching step has been the recent official approval of the drug Lithium carbonate for the treatment of manic-depressive disease. The interest in this carbonated form of the element Lithium is both theoretical and practical. In very small quantities Lithium is present in the human body, in ordinary water and in higher quantity in a number of mineral waters. Lithium affects, among other things, the salt metabolism of the body and in an indirect way those nerve impulse transmissions which were discussed in the chapter on schizophrenia. What may be of the greatest importance is the fact that Lithium seems to be a truly specific treatment of the manic phase of manic-depressive disease. It has very little or no effect on other states of excitement. Furthermore in some manic-depressive patients it acts as a preventive of both manic and depressed phases if taken permanently, and thus is of course of immeasurable value. However, Lithium is not a harmless drug and its administration has to be constantly supervised. Frequent blood samples have to be checked regularly for Lithium concentration in the blood, and one has to watch out for side effects such as nausea, diarrhea, tremor of the hands and edema of the ankles.

Antidepressive Drugs:

There are several types of drugs capable of relieving depression. Drugs containing Dexedrine are rarely used. They have undesirable side effects and are habit forming. Taken in excessive dosages, they can produce an acute brain syndrome. Other antidepressive drugs are of different chemical structures but their common physiological and clinical significance is their ability to act as stimulants or energizers. Probably the site of their action is the hypothalamic area of the brain. The most important of these drugs is imipramine (Tofranil).

TARGET SYMPTOMS AND LIMITATIONS

Target symptoms for these drugs are depressions of the reactive or neurotic, the manic-depressive and the involutional type. Depression with admixtures of schizophrenic elements and particularly schizophrenias of the schizo-affective type are singularly unresponsive to treatment with presently available antidepressive drugs. However, it can be expected that eventually the pharmaceutical industry will find drugs effective in these particular clinical syndromes. Most likely their chemical structure will differ from those of the drugs now in use. Another limitation of the antidepressive drugs is their relatively slow mode of action. Responses cannot ordinarily be observed before the second week of treatment. This constitutes a serious drawback in cases of depressions with suicidal tendencies and in others where for one reason or another treatment has to be completed as quickly as possible. Further, a number of physical ailments, such as high blood pressure and liver and blood diseases, may prohibit the use of one or the other of these drugs.

What has been said about the dangerous side effects of the tranquilizers is equally true for the antidepressants, which in some instances have been proven to be more dangerous than the tranquilizers. It would be a serious mistake to believe that in the treatment of depressions it is safer to use drugs than electroshock therapy. The opposite is true. A number of deaths clearly attributable to the use of these drugs have been reported in the medical literature. The widespread tranquilizing and energizing that is going on throughout our country is not as innocuous as it may seem. However, used wisely in well selected cases and with proper precautions, these drugs are of great value.

Electroconvulsive Therapy:

In 1935, two observations led to the discovery of the convulsive therapies. First, it was thought that epilepsy and schizophrenia were antagonistic and thus could not coexist in the same individual. Furthermore, it had been noticed that schizophrenics suffering isolated spontaneous convulsions improved symptomatically. Taking his cues from such observations, von Meduna in 1935 induced epileptic convulsions in schizophrenic patients by means of chemical agents. In 1938, this method was replaced by U. Cerletti's and L. Bini's simpler and less traumatic electrical provocation of seizures. This method has been standardized and is now being used throughout the world.

The technique consists of applying two electrodes to the temple of the head and sending through the brain an alternate current of about 120 volts for 0.5 to 1 second. The procedure is painless. The patient loses consciousness immediately, has a *grand mal* seizure and regains consciousness within one or two minutes. The seizure is usually followed by normal sleep of one or two hours, after which the patient awakens alert and refreshed. He has no recollection of the treatment.

Like almost any other effective treatment in medicine, electroconvulsive therapy can produce complications, but with sound clinical judgment and good technique they can be reduced to a minimum. Electroconvulsive therapy is a recognized and reasonably safe procedure. One complication, due to the forward bending during the convulsion, is compression of a lumbar vertebra. These compressions are usually mild and do not require treatment, bed rest, or discontinuation of treatment. Severe fractures of the vertebrae or of extremities are very rare and with modern techniques can almost always be avoided. Cardiovascular and respiratory complications are unusual in unmodified electroconvulsive therapy.

Modifications of this form of treatment have been attempted along different avenues. There were attempts to reduce the electric current in order to produce short periods of unconsciousness without convulsions. This proved to be ineffective, however, and it is now recognized that the convulsion is the necessary curative element of the treatment method. Efforts were also made to minimize or abolish the outward manifestations of the convulsion, i.e., the muscular contractions responsible for most of the complications. This was achieved by the administration of the Indian arrow poison, curare, which temporarily blocks the nerve at the site where it penetrates, paralyzing the muscle. There are a number of related drugs now being used in conjunction with electroshock therapy and they are indicated whenever complications from the muscular contractions are anticipated. Whether or not they should be used in other cases as well is a matter of choice. These medications have added to the hazards of the treatment and most of the rare but serious complications are probably due to excessive or imprudent use of these drugs, particularly in conjunction with barbiturates and phenothiazines.

Often, electroconvulsive therapy is viewed by the public and by some physicians as a crude—not to say cruel—and hazardous treatment, apt to cripple the patient's mind and helping only temporarily, if it helps at all. This is a gross and unfortunate misconception. Statistically, electroconvulsive therapy has been shown to be a most successful therapeutic tool when applied with discrimination. Its therapeutic effectiveness is no more and no less "temporary" than any other treatment method which could be used whenever electroconvulsive therapy is indicated. More probably than not, the total number of serious complications due to electroshock treatment during the thirty years of its existence is smaller than the total number of those caused by tranquilizers and anti-depressive drugs during their fifteen year history. Electroconvulsive therapy does indeed produce a certain loss of memory, but this is temporary and does not persist for more than a few weeks. Furthermore, the temporary loss of memory can be minimized by the application of what is called "unilateral" electroshock, whereby both electrodes are placed on the side of the non-dominant hemisphere of the brain. The risk involved in any method of medical treatment has to be balanced against the risk inherent in the disease to be treated. The general practitioner would rarely use general anesthesia for the removal of a toenail, but an inflamed appendix has to be removed by surgical procedure at the risk of serious complications inherent in the nature of the intervention. It would be misleading to minimize the dangers of certain mental diseases and to aggrandize the hazards of some forms of treatment. Psychotic depressions, catatonic states, and extreme forms of manic excitement do threaten the life of the patient and have to be treated quickly and effectively. Electroconvulsive therapy can be life- and agony-saving in all three of these conditions.

Indications:

Electroshock treatment was conceived as a specific therapy for schizophrenia but quickly it proved to be more effective in depressions than in schizophrenia. The most responsive target symptom for this treatment, therefore, is the psychotic depression. Catatonic symptoms usually react favorably and so do schizophrenic symptoms of the schizo-affective type. For the most part, manic excitement can be controlled with phenothiazines, but occasionally electroconvulsive therapy is unavoidable and it is successful.

As a general rule, it can be said that electroconvulsive therapy is maximally effective in acute psychotic conditions marked by depression or catatonic symptomatology or by other manifestations of severe anxiety and tension. Neuroses, character disorder, paranoid conditions, simple and other chronic forms of schizophrenia do not respond favorably to electroshock therapy. It is rarely indicated in acute or chronic brain syndromes.

Nothing has been said about the way in which electroconvulsive treatment brings about its curative effects because nothing definite is known about it. The interested reader will find theoretical discussions of the subject in the appropriate textbooks.

There are other forms of somatic treatment, such as insulin coma therapy and prefrontal lobotomy or psychosurgery, that are indicated in some cases. They play a minor role in present day psychiatry, and will not be discussed.

PSYCHOLOGICAL TREATMENT

Introductory Remarks:

Definition: By the general term "psychological treatment" we mean any goal-directed attempt by a skilled therapist to influence his patient's psyche, feelings, attitude, and behavior by psychological methods. This can be accomplished through individual or group psychotherapy, through psychodrama, psychosocial counseling, or through the establishment of a therapeutic ward milieu.

Psychological treatment can be of a covering or uncovering nature. The covering methods do not try to provide the patient with deep insight and understanding of his emotional problems. They attempt to reorient him, through such methods as persuasion, hypnosis, and reconditioning. The uncovering or analytical methods strive to get at the root of the psychological conflicts and to make the patient understand them. To reach this goal, a variety of techniques have been devised, based on different schools of thought.

The goal of psychological therapy cannot be stated in a simple sentence. It can be the abolishment of a hysterical paralysis of the right hand by means of a single hypnotic session, and in this the therapist may be successful. It can be the complete analysis, reorientation, and readaptation to life of a psychoneurotic by means of four analytical hours per week for five years, and the therapist may fail. Like the goals of somatic therapy, those of psychological treatment must be flexible and relative, realistically taking into account the potentials and limitations of the patient and the method. The power of psychological therapy has been both grossly under- and overestimated. For many people, analytical psychotherapy has come to represent a mystical, all-powerful key to every emotional problem, unlocking the secrets of men's psychoses. Nothing of the sort can be expected.

Some believe that what man really is lies hidden under the surface of his obvious personality and that scratching at this surface will uncover his true self. What has so frequently and blissfully been called "depth-analysis" is in many instances no more than scratching the surface, even when it unearths what are supposed to have been the patient's feelings at age three. Man is not so much what he hides as what he makes of himself; not so much his unconscious as his conscious existence. His "surface" is the end result of his efforts to integrate a multitude of strivings and reactions, of needs and impressions, and as such it is the essence of him. Every wise man has overcome foolishness within himself, as every saint has overcome evil, and it is meaningless to say that the wise man is "really" a fool, and the saint "basically" a sinner. Certainly improvement of the surface can constitute a therapeutic goal, but the complexity of the growth process limits the remodeling possibilities.

Adjustment has been called a therapeutic goal. But adjustment to what? The goal of psychotherapy may well be nonadjustment, if adjustment were to signify death of individuality. Many other lofty concepts have been declared goals of psychotherapy, but to the author it would seem more realistic to envisage partial and specific goals rather than global and vague ones. In psychological therapy as in any other medical therapy, compensation of function may be the key word. Basic to any kind of psychological treatment are the search for patterns of behavior that disturb the proper functioning of the individual, an attempt to understand their origin as far as possible and to correct them. To make this possible, a good emotional relationship between patient and therapist is a prerequisite; not only will it help the patient to bare his innermost feelings and thoughts, but it will show him also that trusting others is possible, and that to have compassion may still be a worthwhile experience.

Indications for psychological treatment in one form or another exist in almost all mentally ill persons, even when the illness itself, the somatic process, cannot be altered by psychological means. A goal-directed plan as to how to approach a patient, what to discuss with him, and where to help him must be an integrated part of every treatment plan. Physician, social worker, and nurses work together with the patient and his family in an attempt to create optimal conditions for the improvement of the illness and the stabilization of the home situation.

Beyond this, the more specific psychotherapeutic methods, like individual and group therapy, are indicated wherever definite emotional problems and conflicts are a part of the illness. This can be the case in a patient with schizophrenia or with manic-depressive disease, in an elderly person with a beginning chronic brain syndrome, or in a psychopath.

Strictly analytical psychotherapies are used in psycho-neuroses. They are not indicated in most psychotic conditions. As to the brand of analytical therapy one should choose, the author can only state that in his opinion this is immaterial. What cures or helps is the personality and the skill of the therapist, not his method or his creed.

In individual psychotherapy the therapist sees one patient at regular intervals. The therapy can be of the covering or the uncovering type or it can be eclectic, i.e., combining various elements from different therapeutic methods. It can consist of a few sessions or can extend over a number of years. It has been declared with assurance that some persons need four years of intensive analytical psychotherapy. Individual psychotherapy can be an extremely stimulating experience for the patient as well as for the therapist, but equally it can develop into a meaningless and sterile "going over the past." If in psychotherapy the patient experiences nothing of significance within six months, it might be appropriate to change the therapist or to discontinue therapy altogether.

In group psychotherapy one or several therapists see from eight to twelve patients in one session. The therapist serves as a stimulator, catalyst, and coordinator for the patients, who speak freely about their personal problems, criticizing, supporting, attacking, and analyzing each other. In all this they are apt to do a thorough job. It is a fascinating experience to observe how each participant is gradually drawn into the general discussion, learning about others and about himself, gradually realizing that his difficulties are not as unique as he thought them to be, and learning how others handle what he could not.

In psychodrama a number of patients stage impromptu sketches of key issues in the life of one or the other of them. The therapist guides the sessions, which in many ways emulate in more plastic fashion the processes of group psychotherapy.

Psychosocial Therapy:

Under this term we group all those activities geared toward helping the patient with whatever social problems he may have. This is primarily the field of the social worker. Rarely, we have said, is mental illness the result of social situations as such, but few will doubt that an unfortunate environment can participate in bringing on mental illness and in perpetuating it. Thus, a clash with superiors over deteriorating performance at work is more likely to be the result of a beginning mental illness than the cause of it. Similar situations arise at home, as we have seen in the case study of the woman with the brain tumor. The patient under treatment must either remain in his environment or return to it eventually. The relatives or the boss at the job need to be properly informed as to the nature of the conflict that led to difficulties. This will relieve anger and possible guilt feelings, bring about better relationships, and improve the chances of maintaining the improvement in the patient's condition brought about by other means.

THE SOCIAL WORKER

The social worker's task is a delicate and important one. Starting with the first contact he has to gain the confidence of the patient and the patient's relatives. Subsequently, he may have to spend much time with some relatives who need reassurance, explanations, and an understanding of their own as well as of the patient's conflicts, shortcomings, and prejudices. He may have to make home visits, to see parents or a spouse who refuse to come to the hospital, or to get a personal view of what the home situation of his patient is like. He may also assemble a number of parents and spouses of patients and have group therapy sessions with them.

Another aspect of psychosocial therapy is the social rehabilitation of the chronic patient who is ready to leave the hospital, but may be reluctant to do so, or may have no home, no relatives, and no job. Placement in foster homes, supervision while in foster homes, and help in finding work or shelter are part of this task.

The social worker plays an equally important role in keeping the released patient out of the hospital. Only a small proportion of all released patients continue to take medication and have to see the physician; others are followed, supported, and helped along by the social worker alone. The social worker will alert the physician when changes in the patient warrant a visit with the doctor, reinstitution of medication, or other measures.

Management of the Schizophrenic Patient:

In applying what we have learned about mental disorders and management, we can now state that, for instance, there is no specific treatment plan for "schizophrenia." Although it is possible to establish certain general patterns for therapy and their results, it remains necessary to approach each patient as an individual, with his personal problems, peculiarities, and as it were his particular "brand of schizophrenia."

Over a period of years or decades, the schizophrenic process waxes and wanes, is acute, chronic, phasic, or continuous. Each stage needs its proper attention and care. At one time the patient may be treated at home, in a doctor's office, or in an outpatient clinic; at another, he may need to interrupt his work and attend a day hospital. Finally, there may come a time when he has to be hospitalized, either on a voluntary basis or by court commitment. It is easy to see that somatic, psychological, and psychosocial therapies have to be applied in ever-changing patterns to fit the momentary and long-range needs of the patient.

The principles guiding the management of the schizophrenic patient may be summarized as follows: reduce or eliminate acute psychopathology, such as anxiety, tension, excitement, delusions, and hallucinations. This is best done by means of adequate doses of phenothiazine tranquilizers or electroconvulsive therapy. Further, treat the remaining strength of the patient, try to split off the sick part of him, counteract his tendency to withdraw, and encourage social activities. See to it that the patient lives a well-regulated but active life. In those cases we cannot cure, we must attempt to retain an optimal level of compensation outside the hospital. We must equally realize that in possibly one third of all cases the price of keeping a patient in the community can become too high in frustration, disruption, and unhappiness, for the patient as well as for those who have to live with him. These patients are better off in hospitals.

Outlook:

If we now pass in review the needs of the mentally ill, as demonstrated in the example of the schizophrenic patient, we must come to the conclusion that more often than not mental illness is a long-term problem. As the patient shifts back and forth through the various phases of health, illness, and functional compensation, so do his psychiatric and psychosocial needs. How well are we presently equipped to provide for these needs and what changes and improvements might be suggested?

As it should be, a large proportion of the mentally ill are being cared for by the general practitioner; a decidedly smaller one by private psychiatrists. If hospitalization becomes necessary, private hospitals are available as well as psychiatric sections in many general hospitals. Usually as a last and desperate step, commitment to a public mental hospital is considered. Private care is expensive and in most cases has to be paid for by the patient or his family. Mental hospitals are often located in isolated areas, many are inadequate and all are understaffed. Outpatient facilities are now provided by mental hygiene clinics and some general and university hospitals. They too are inadequate. Worse, there is little cohesion among all these facilities, which usually are located far apart from one another. The hospital doctor rarely hears what the general practitioner has observed and prescribed, and in most instances the general practitioner or private psychiatrist has only a vague report on the proceedings in the hospital. Over the years, the patient himself may well visit a good number of different facilities and each time speak to a doctor he has never seen before, who has little or no knowledge of which treatment methods had already been discarded as ineffective and which had been found useful. To be sure, each doctor or social worker involved does his best to help, but as a whole the procedure is unsatisfactory and, in part, disgraceful.

During the past few years, much thinking and experimenting has been done in an attempt to conceptualize better ways of caring for the mentally ill. In several papers F. A. Freyhan and J. Mayo* have presented a well considered model for a modern comprehensive psychiatric center. In the remaining part of this chapter the author will essentially follow their concept.

Any such model has to consist of several units, namely: a hospital for inpatient care; a day hospital, in which patients can be treated during the day, staying at home at night; an outpatient clinic; a home service; and various community facilities, such as foster homes and half-way houses. For therapeutic and administrative reasons, the various components of the center should form a single unit with regard to location and staffing. Such a center would have cohesion in purpose and action, and the difficulties mentioned above could be avoided or minimized.

In cities, a mental hospital, if located within easy reach of the community it serves, or a sufficiently large and independent wing of a general hospital, should serve as headquarters for the comprehensive psychiatric center. Within its building or within a reasonable distance from it

*F. A. Freyhan and J. Mayo, "Concept of a Model Psychiatric Clinic." *American Journal of Psychiatry* September 1963, and "A Comprehensive Psychiatric Center," U. S. Department of Health, Education, and Welfare, 1963.

should be located the day hospital and the outpatient clinic. The same medical, social service, and administrative staff would be responsible for all facilities. A home service, composed of doctors, social workers, and nurses, would be available to all units. Consultants in various specialties and the private psychiatrists and general practitioners of the community should all be intimately involved in this treatment center.

A patient should be able to come to the center on his own, as a referral by an outside physician, or by court commitment. On arrival, he and his responsible relatives would be interviewed by an evaluating team of physicians and social workers, and if necessary emergency tests would be performed, such as electroencephalograms or psychological tests. According to the decision of the evaluation team, it would be suggested to the patient that he either start treatment in the outpatient clinic, come to the day hospital, or enter the hospital as an inpatient.

Comprehensive evaluation and treatment in the hospital should be well focused, prompt, and, hopefully, short. As soon as the patient's condition permits, he should move into the day hospital, where active therapy will continue. The day hospital must have a well-regulated and stimulating therapeutic program and the patient's stay in it should be limited to about two months. It is in operation during regular working hours and the participating patients are required to attend regularly. The day hospital should not become a clubhouse or waiting room where former patients may or may not spend their idle time.

As a next step, the patient might attend the outpatient clinic. There he may receive drugs, participate in individual or group psychotherapy, or in counseling sessions with a social worker. If he is well enough, he should cease to be an outpatient, but at any time he should be able to return there for further help, which may consist of short counseling, renewed drug treatment, or referral to the day hospital or the general hospital.

The home service team visits patients in their homes. The purpose of such a visit may be a re-evaluation of the patient's situation, emergency treatment, or the administration of drug or psychological therapy.

The advantages of such a comprehensive psychiatric center are self-evident. Hopefully, without therapeutic bias and in close contact with the community it serves, it not only is able to render maximal help to its patients, but also to serve as an ideal center for research and training.

·VIII·

Psychiatry and the Law

A book such as this can only touch on some of the basic issues that arise when the mentally ill are confronted with legal procedures. In legal terms, mental illness is referred to as *insanity,* and psychiatry dealing with questions of law is called *forensic psychiatry.*

Naturally, both lawyers and psychiatrists are concerned with human behavior but tend to look at it from different angles. Whereas the psychiatrist is used to perceive behavior as the result of often unconscious, or conditioned, psychological dynamics and motivations, and is trained rather to understand than to moralize, the jurist

213

judges behavior on the basis of certain generalized rules which apply to the average man and society as a whole. He assumes free will much more readily than do psychiatrists. From this, numerous misunderstandings and often acrimonious debates between psychiatrists and lawyers derive, as well as the distaste of many psychiatrists to testify in court and the impatience of lawyers with the often longwinded and tortuous arguments of some psychiatrists. There remains much to be learned on both sides of the fence, since, actually, there should not be a fence at all; lawyers and psychiatrists should work together in harmony for the benefit of the individual and society at large. It must be said, however, that in this respect much effort and progress has been made in various judicial districts within the United States.

At its most dramatic, the issue of insanity is frequently raised in cases of murder. The recent past has provided us with a sad number of spectacular single, often political or multiple murders, in which a person with zeal and persistence stalks his victim across the country, or in a sudden frenzy shoots wildly and indiscriminately at anyone who happens to be around at the particular moment.

What, then, are the basic problems we have to discuss in such cases? Obviously, mental disorder as such does not spell lack of criminal responsibility, as it is called. A paranoid schizophrenic who functions quite well in many of his activities and may even hold a job to his employer's satisfaction, may on his way to the office fail to stop at a red light and hit another car. Most likely his paranoid ideas have nothing to do with this accident and the question of insanity will not come up. However, suppose this same man drives on a highway, sees another car follow him and believes that it must belong to one of his fancied enemies, "out to get him." He slows down, lets the other car pass and then forces him off the road, thereby killing the driver. He obviously is acting in accordance with his delusions. Here insanity becomes an issue.

Thus the crucial question concerns the more or less intimate connection between the criminal act and the state of mental illness of the offender. In some cases this will be crystal clear to everyone concerned, possibly with the exception of the mentally ill himself. In other instances such a connection may be obscure and hotly debated between prosecution and defense. Both will then call on psychiatrists to examine the accused and testify in court as to his mental condition. Yet the issues may be so involved that even the psychiatrists among themselves come to different conclusions. Usually the questions addressed to the psychiatrist are these: was the offender capable of forming an intent to commit the act in question? Has the defendant's mental condition been such that he was, at the time of the offense, able or unable to distinguish between right and wrong, and if he was able to do so, was he able or unable to adhere to the right, or was he, for example, acting on the basis of an irresistible impulse?

A man with an organic brain disorder, let us say with a tumor of the forebrain, may be so confused mentally that he no longer realizes the wrongness of exposing his genitals in front of a young girl in a park. In another instance, a sexual psychopath may very well know all the legal consequences of such an act, but may nevertheless have such a strong, irresistible impulse to expose himself that he cannot refrain from doing so. Finally, the above mentioned paranoid driver may be perfectly aware of his criminal intent but his delusional thinking may dictate to him: "He will kill me unless I get him first," and he will act accordingly.

If the insanity is so manifest as in the first and the last cases, the issues may not be difficult to decide. However, much more critical, intricate and debatable are the questions involving irresistible impulse. Here the examination of the offender must be exceedingly critical and the decision whether or not one is dealing with a truly irresistible impulse may in the last analysis rest with the credibility of the offender and the personal, subjective conviction of the psychiatrist.

The laws governing these issues vary greatly from one country to another and, within the United States, from one state to another. In some countries the courts will rule by a simple scale of yes or no, in others they recognize graduations and speak, for example, of diminution of responsibility, even to the extent of percentages of such a diminution according to the degree of impairment of mental functions.

Obviously, the mentally ill offender will not be helped by imprisonment or other punitive measures. What he needs is psychiatric assistance, and as enlightenment in this area as well as proper facilities for such cases increase, he is more frequently getting it. But here, too, actual practices vary greatly and are presently much debated.

Many unresolved and vexing problems surround court procedures and sentencing or commitment to institutions of the so-called criminally insane. For once, the responsibility for the release from the psychiatric hospital of a court-committed murderer or rapist rests with the superintendent of the hospital. How sure can he ever be that his patient is really cured and, once released, will not commit another offense? With the sexual psychopath or the paranoid schizophrenic, this can be extremely difficult to decide and honest misjudgments can and do occur.

Also it goes without saying that an acutely schizophrenic or manic person who has committed a crime during his psychosis and has subsequently been committed to a hospital for therapy may have genuinely recovered and be ready for discharge in a relatively short time. Had he not been mentally ill and committed the same offense, he might remain in prison for many years. This may move a defense lawyer to plead insanity for his client even when this is hardly warranted.

Questions of mental health and illness play a role not only in criminal law but in civil law as well. For example, the issue of insanity may be raised in instances involving irresponsible financial transactions, the signing of deeds, annulment and divorce or the drawing of a will. Last but not least there is the whole issue of legal commitment of a mentally ill person to a psychiatric hospital in the absence of any legal offense. Often such a commitment entails the temporary loss of certain civil rights, such as the writing of checks, voting, making legally binding decisions and so forth. Unless the mentally ill is assumed to be dangerous to others or to himself and nevertheless refuses to enter a hospital, the present tendency is to refrain from legal commitment whenever possible, i.e., to encourage and persuade the patient to enter the hospital voluntarily. Also, legal commitment can be divorced from the loss of civil rights, as is the case now in the District of Columbia. The interested reader will find more information on these matters in books on forensic psychiatry (see Bibliography).

·IX·

Mental Illness in the United States

The Magnitude of the Problem:

The magnitude of the problem posed by mental illness in terms of individual and collective sorrow, stress, and financial burden can be demonstrated in various ways. Statistics are indispensable, but not always reliable. For instance, the number of yearly admissions to public mental hospitals in the United States can be correctly determined. But one can only estimate the amount of money that the mentally ill, were they sane, would contribute to the national income. Statistics need interpretation to become meaningful. Thus, whether or not first-admission rates to mental hospitals within a given area permit conclusions as to the extent of mental illness in that area will depend on a variety of factors. For instance,

218

we know that admission rates in India cannot be compared with those in the United States since in India the number of available hospital beds is hopelessly inadequate, whereas in the United States it is not. But even where hospital beds are available, admission rates will depend on the existence and efficiency of psychiatric outpatient services in general hospitals and on community mental health clinics. Admission rates will also depend on the number and availability of psychiatrists and the willingness of general practitioners to treat mental patients. Finally, one cannot overlook such factors as the readiness of the population to commit sick relatives to mental hospitals, or their ability to manage the sick at home. In rural communities these situations may differ very much from those in cities. To illustrate, in the state of New Mexico there are 116 hospitalized mental patients per 100,000 population, as against 585 in New York State (1956). It is hardly permissible to conclude that the New Mexicans are healthier than the New Yorkers. Only if it were possible to take into account all these and other factors would admission rates to mental hospitals become meaningful with respect to the extent of mental illness in a given area.

Other figures in need of interpretation are those concerned with hospital discharges. For instance, would an increase in discharges mean that therapy had become more effective? Certainly, such a conclusion could not be arrived at without a very close scrutiny of the discharge policies involved. There have been times when psychiatrists were most reluctant to discharge patients showing such mild remnants of disease as occasional hallucinations or odd behavior. The consequences were long periods of hospitalization, relatively few discharges and increase in hospital populations. Presently, thinking and policies in this respect are undergoing marked changes. It is felt that hospitalization ought to be short; that the patient, once over the acuteness of his illness, should return home and complete his treatment as an outpatient. Also, psychiatrists today are less concerned over a patient's continuing to show some signs of his illness as long as he makes an acceptable adjustment in the community, and as long as the community accepts him as he is.

With regard to statistics, such policies cause a shortening of hospitalization for many patients, and an increase in discharge rates. They also lead to an increase in the numbers of readmissions, since not all patients remain well. Does all this mean that treatment has improved? Perhaps, but there is much disagreement over this point, some arguing that therapy should be called unsuccessful unless it brings about complete cure. At this point, however, we are concerned with showing the need for interpretation of statistics and not with the results of such interpretations.

Quite apart from statistics, but equally part of the magnitude of the problem of mental illness, is an entirely different set of circumstances which remain elusive and not susceptible to statistical treatment. At best, they may be gauged by empathy and estimate. We are speaking of the impact the mentally ill often have on their family and community in terms of emotional stress and worry, despair, and disruption, and financial expenses. It is easy to exaggerate such influences but hard to deny them altogether. There are families, industrious, proud, and ambitious, who completely falter when mental illness strikes. Others, once they have hospitalized the sick relative, close ranks and try to live on as if there had never been a casualty. However, guilt feelings, more or less unconscious, may color and plague their thoughts and actions for a long time to come. There are powerful, effective, and creative citizens who, at the height of their careers, become mentally ill without ever recovering entirely. And, there are the poor who, if they become ill early, may for the rest of their lives remain a financial burden to the community.

At the time of the original publication of this book in 1963, the United States was in a rather unique position, inasmuch as it had just been presented with the findings of a detailed survey of its entire mental health problems. It is appropriate to relate briefly how this came about.

During the past fifty years the general population of the United States has doubled. The mental hospital population, however, has quadrupled. The professional staff available to take care of this ever-increasing number of patients became entirely inadequate. Thus, in 1954 there were individual state mental hospitals in the United States with as many as 15,000 inmates, with an often inadequately-trained psychiatrist trying to attend to the needs of 400 and more patients. There were mental hospitals housing together almost 40,000 patients without a psychiatrist on the staff. One dollar per mental patient was spent yearly for research in the field of psychiatry, as against $900 for poliomyelitis. The mentally ill, although occupying one out of every two hospital beds in the United States, were thoroughly neglected and frequently almost forgotten.

Upon the urging of some of the leading psychiatrists of the country, Congress finally passed the Mental Health Act of 1955, charging the National Institute of Mental Health with the task of analyzing all problems involving mental illness and health in the United States and submitting recommendations for improvement. The Joint Commission on Mental Illness and Health was formed, composed of physicians, psychologists, anthropologists, educators, clergymen, administrators, and many others. In December, 1960, the Commission presented its findings and recommendations in a voluminous final report: *Action for Mental Health.* Subsequently, the President of the United States sent a message to Congress outlining the need and urgency for legislative action in this entire area of mental illness and mental deficiency.

Undoubtedly, the report and the President's message have favorably affected the management of the mentally ill in the United States. The main theme of decentralization of care, with emphasis on new community treatment centers and psychiatric facilities in general hospitals, together with shorter hospitalization periods, has been successfully pursued up to a point. This is discussed more comprehensively in the chapter on management. Presently, i.e., in 1972, some of the original enthusiasm is in danger of slacking. Difficulties in the financing, locating, staffing and managing of these community centers have arisen, and a good deal of rethinking of these matters is in progress. This is unavoidable of course, whenever new avenues of exploration in a given field are searched for.

However, at this point we have to return to statistics and to some of the findings of the Joint Commission. Having read so much about the various mental illnesses, the reader no doubt would like to know how many mentally ill persons there are in the United States.

Unfortunately, this question is difficult to answer. It has been suggested that in the United States one out of ten persons will at one time or another during his lifetime need treatment for emotional illness. Such a figure is meaningless. It raises a host of hotly debated issues, such as: Who needs psychiatric treatment? Do all those who seek treatment need it? Should some or many of those who do not look for therapy receive it? What, really, is meant by psychiatric treatment? Is a single therapeutic discussion between patient and internist on the emotional background of a heart attack considered psychiatric treatment? Repeated dialogues with a minister, resulting in the salvaging of a marriage, are they not psychiatric treatment? And finally, what is meant by these terms "mental illness" or "mental disorders," as they are generally used? There is little agreement on this issue. And even if there were agreement, could all mentally ill persons be accounted for? For instance, it is likely but not certain that schizophrenics, manic-depressives, and persons with senile brain disorders will be hospitalized at least once during their lifetime. With moderate accuracy, these can be accounted for. But who could ever hope to estimate the number of psychoneurotics or persons with character disorders, who rarely enter mental hospitals? The reader will do well to bear such reservations in mind in the following accounts, and in others like them.

In 1961, there were in the United States 286 public mental hospitals and 276 private mental hospitals. A quickly increasing number (598) of psychiatric facilities in general hospitals have had to be added. Together these hospitals provided approximately 800,000 beds.* (The total number of hospital beds in the United States is

*These figures do not include hospitals reserved for mentally defectives. However, many mentally defectives reside in the above-cited public hospitals.

1,612,822.) Despite their small number of beds, the general hospitals and particularly the private hospitals have relatively higher admission and discharge rates than do the public mental hospitals. This is understandable, since in these facilities the cost of maintenance and care is high and treatment is thus reserved primarily for acute conditions.

The following tables will give an impression of the admission and discharge rates of public mental hospitals, the size of the hospital population and their composition according to diagnoses.

To the numbers of the mentally ill treated as in-patients, we have to add the growing number of those who are being cared for as outpatients. Figures illustrating this concern the mental health clinics that exist in all parts of the country.

TABLE I

Yearly Admission and Discharge Rates in Public Mental Hospitals in the U. S. A.				
	1950	1956	1959	1971
All Admissions	152,286	185,597	223,225	414,926
First Admissions	114,054	125,539	142,881	*
Readmissions	38,232	60,058	80,344	*
Discharges	99,659	145,208	176,411	*
Patients residing in hospital at end of year	512,501	551,390	541,883	338,592
Annual maintenance expense per residing patient	$ 779.61	$1,195.01	$1,567.39	$6,420.00

*Due to different data collections, comparable 1971 figures are not available. The figures in this table and the following pages were provided by the office for statistics, American Psychiatric Association, Washington, D. C.

What can be seen in Table I is a significant shift around the year 1956. Although total admissions, first admissions and readmissions continue to rise, the number of patients residing in hospitals at any given time declined drastically. This trend coincided with the introduction of psychopharmacological treatment methods, i.e., tranquilizers and antidepressant drugs, and the ensuing liberalization of ideas about necessity of hospitalization and the build-up of outpatient treatment. This trend continues.

TABLE II

Composition According to Diagnosis of Admissions (1969)

Total Admissions: 367,963

Schizophrenias	100,398 (27.2%)
Alcoholic Disorders	94,589 (25.7%)
Organic Brain Syndrome	39,831 (10.8%)
Psychoneuroses	31,264 (8.5%)
Personality Disorders	27,315 (7.4%)
Affective Disorders	13,553 (3.7%)
(manic-depressive disease and other depressions)	
Other Psychoses	12,048 (3.3%)
Drug Disorders	10,531 (2.9%)
Mental Retardation	9,897 (2.7%)
All Other Disorders	28,537 (7.8%)

In 1956, 1,294 mental health clinics treated 380,000 patients. In 1961 there were already 1,600 mental health clinics taking care of 665,000 patients. In 1969 there were nearly 2,400 mental health clinics serving about 1,900,000 persons. These clinics usually have a rapid turnover.

Originally, most patients were seen for evaluation, and only about one-third of them received treatment. Continuous increase in the number of these clinics and a change in their pattern toward greater treatment orientation will further improve their usefulness (See Chapter VII).

A few words should be said about the cost involved in the care of the mentally ill. In his message to Congress, in February of 1963, the President specified that care of the mentally ill cost the taxpayers $2.4 billion yearly in direct public outlay for services. Indirect public outlay, including welfare costs and such, would be much higher. The state of New York, for instance, assigns 10 per cent of its annual budget to matters concerning mental illness.

The growing concern with mental illness and health is well illustrated by the increasing appropriations made by Congress to the National Institute of Mental Health.

TABLE III

Appropriations of the U. S. Congress for major activities of the National Institutes of Health. (In millions of dollars.)

	1956	1964	1970
Cancer	18.9	145.1	190.4
Heart Diseases	10.7	133.6	171.3
Mental Health	8.7	180.0	358.4

With these appropriations the National Institute of Mental Health finances research programs within their own walls at Bethesda, Maryland, and also sponsors and supports other research conducted in hospitals and institutions throughout the country. It contributes to training programs for professional staffs and to a great variety of other activities designed to improve mental health in the United States and abroad.

Finally, there are data, some accurate, some estimates, which may involve mental illness in more indirect ways. Here we think of the estimated 21,325 suicides per year (1967), or 10.8 suicides per 100,000 population; the 13,425 homicides, or 6.8 per 100,000 population for 1967; the estimated 10 million alcoholics (1972), and the 660,000 marriages that ended in divorce in 1969. Such figures, in one way or another, reflect human tragedies. Suicide, in our opinion, is not necessarily a sign of mental imbalance or mental illness. Nevertheless, more often than not it will be the result of emotional turmoil and often it is the final action of a person with a serious depression. Homicides are committed by supposedly perfectly normal people, but for the most part they are the acts of warped minds, but warped not necessarily in the sense of a psychosis. As a matter of fact, the notorious "madman," the psychotic schizophrenic or manic, is rarely the perpetrator of serious crimes. A problem drinker is understood to be a person who, on account of emotional difficulties, cannot control his drinking and thus causes hardship and harm to himself and his family. There are a number of alcoholics who enter and remain in mental hospitals, at the expected height of their occupational careers, because of the irreparable damage done to their brains. Divorce is sometimes due to the mental illness and prolonged hospitalization of a spouse.

As an interesting aside, statistics clearly indicate that single persons have much higher admission rates to mental institutions than do married persons, regardless of age, sex, or diagnosis. This significant finding needs interpretation. Persons who become mentally ill later in their lives often have character traits that made them unsuitable for marriage. If mental illness strikes early in life, the former patient, once recovered, is less likely to marry than a person who has never been mentally ill. However, he remains apt to have recurrences of his illness. Older single people, particularly women during the years of their menopause, tend to feel lonely and depressed. Since often they have nobody to take care of them, they need hospitalization. Marriage, on the other hand, seems to have certain protective qualities by providing goals, responsibilities, and satisfactions. If one spouse takes ill, the other will care for him or her at home if at all possible. The responsibility and necessity to provide for a family may keep a married man at his job as long as he can function, whereas a single person, having to care only for himself, may give up earlier. Finally, when old age causes mental deterioration, children sometimes take care of the parent, whereas the single person may have no alternative to hospitalization.

Mental Illness in Other Countries:

In reviewing psychiatric problems in countries around the globe, we must distinguish between two aspects, namely, the existence, form, and content of mental disorders, and the manner in which the mentally ill are taken care of. We will briefly discuss these problems.

The idea is sometimes advanced that as to their mind, psyche, or psychological development and reactions, men differ so much from one another that they can never be compared, that their mental disorders cannot be classified and that their treatment must be strictly individualized. However, experience and a view directed not so much to details as to the overall design of human affairs would seem to point in exactly the opposite direction. Men, so it appears, are much more alike than they are dissimilar. This may displease some who, with regard to man's development in general and the emergence of mental disorders in particular, place great stock in the importance of culture, environment, and family attitudes.

From admittedly incomplete records, one might conclude with fair accuracy that distributions and forms of mental disorders all over the world are similar and comparable. Schizophrenia, for instance, with only minor variations affects as many persons in the European, African, and Asian countries as it does on the American continents. The American or European psychiatrist encounters no difficulty in recognizing schizophrenia in native Africans or Japanese, and his Asian colleagues are well able to use our present classification in diagnosing all mental disorders in their own countries.

There may be regional differences in the incidence of manic-depressive disease, but depressions are a universal phenomenon. Content of psychoses will always depend on personal experience and the surrounding cultural patterns in which the patient has grown up. The neuroses, hysteria in particular, invariably have been more culture-bound in form and temporal incidence than the psychoses. Today, the classical form of hysteria hardly exists as described by Jean Marie Charcot. Emotional problems remain the same, but the behavioral expressions change with time and mores.

Obviously, one must expect differences in the incidence of infections and toxic psychoses according to the level of civilization and available medical facilities. Alcoholism, with all its complications, is little known among Muslims and in other countries where alcohol is against religious beliefs, and some of the intoxicating effects of plants chewed by natives in South America are not seen in the United States.

Although the mentally ill live in all parts of the world, the attention they receive varies greatly from continent to continent. How they are treated will depend on the level of civilization of the country, its economic and social structure, and the availability of professional personnel and appropriate facilities. India in 1963, for instance, had 15,000 hospital beds for the mentally ill, but these beds are "occupied" by 30,000 patients. Actually, it has been estimated that in India there are 2 million persons in need of psychiatric treatment, but there are less than 200 psychiatrists in the entire country, which corresponds to a ratio of 0.3 psychiatrists per 100,000 population (554,600,000). (These and the following figures are from the 1971 Directory of the World Psychiatric Association. "Membership" in societies does not necessarily reflect the number of actually practicing psychiatrists.)

Corresponding figures for the United Kingdom are: 4,450 members of the Psychiatric Association, which equals a rate of 7.9 psychiatrists per 100,000 population (56,000,000). The Federal Republic of Germany has 952 members in its Society for Psychiatry and Neurology, with a rate of 1.6 psychiatrists per 100,000 population (58,600,000), whereas there are 383 members of the corresponding Society in the Democratic Republic of

Germany (East Germany), with a ratio of 2.4 per 100,000 population (16,200,000). For figures for the U. S. see Appendix (pp. 235-236).

Countries like England, Denmark, Norway, and Sweden are pioneering in the management of the mentally ill. In these countries, the pace has been set for such methods as extensive home and family care, early and short treatment in outpatient facilities of general hospitals, in day hospitals and therapeutic communities. England already has reduced the number of its mental hospitals and plans to continue to do so. Whereas in the United States 85 per cent of all patients in mental hospitals are committed there by the court, in England the same percentage applies to voluntary admissions.

In Russia psychiatry is well developed and in many ways progressive in the management of the mentally ill. There are 20,000 psychiatrists, constituting a ratio of 8.2 psychiatrists per 100,000 population (241,748,000). In 1963 there existed only 140,000 mental hospital beds, most patients receiving outpatient treatment in what are called dispensaries. If hospitalization is unavoidable, it is first attempted in a general or specialized psychiatric dispensary which has a few beds for short hospitalization.

How cultural patterns affect psychiatric management problems is well illustrated by the fate of the senile patients in different countries. In the United States these patients pose a tremendous problem because they fill about one third of all beds in mental hospitals and often they stay there for years. In India this problem does not exist since religious traditions make it mandatory for the children to provide for their parents.

A few generalities can be stated: Mental illness is a universal problem. Psychiatric management has undergone profound changes within the last few decades, particularly in the Western Hemisphere and in Russia. In other parts of the world, psychiatry shares the slow process of awakening and progressing civilization. The problems to be conquered are staggering. They concern the training of physicians, nurses, social workers, and psychologists, the building of hospitals and community clinics, and last but not least, the education and enlightenment of the general population with regard to mental illness.

Appendix

THE STAFF OF A MENTAL INSTITUTION

In a modern American mental hospital or mental health clinic a well-established team of specialists usually participates in caring for mental patients. The person in charge is the psychiatrist, although some mental health clinics may not have a psychiatrist as a full-time member on their staff. The social worker and the psychologist work with the psychiatrist. The psychiatric nurse and her aides have the closest and most constant contact with the patient. Added to this basic staff will be found, according to the size and function of the clinic or hospital, occupational, recreational, and dance therapists, and perhaps experts in psychodrama. In the remaining pages we will sketch the training and function of some members of this team.

The Psychiatrist:

The psychiatrist is a physician. After completion of medical school and a one-year internship in a general hospital, he begins special training in psychiatry. For this purpose he enters a psychiatric training center in a university hospital or a state mental hospital. The training center must be approved as such by the American Psychiatric Association and fulfill certain minimum requirements with regard to the provision of a well-rounded theoretical and practical training program for the physician. After completion of this residency, which extends over a period of three years, the psychiatrist can seek further specialization—in child psychiatry or in psychoanalysis, for instance. After two more years of practice in psychiatry, the physician is eligible to take specialty examinations which are provided by the American Board of Psychiatry and Neurology, Inc., a private institution for the safeguarding of psychiatric standards. Board examinations are not compulsory but the majority of newly trained psychiatrists in the United States take them. One can assume that a Board member has fulfilled minimal training requirements, is of good moral standing, and has successfully weathered a full day of rigorous examinations in psychiatry and neurology.

In Great Britain, the training of psychiatrists also ends with stringent Specialty Board examinations. In Germany, however, training seems to be much less structured and regulated, and at this point there are no final specialty examinations. Also, in Germany, there is a rather sharp division between psychiatrists and psychotherapists. The division of the fields of psychiatry and neurology has not yet been formalized, as is the case in the United States. The teaching and practice of psychotherapy and psycho-analysis, which are integral parts of the training of the American and British psychiatrist, are not practiced in Germany, but are left to non-medical professions, such as psychologists and therapists, who are trained as psycho-analysts. In the author's view this is an unfortunate state of affairs. Neurology as well as psychiatry has developed into two vast specialties which can hardly be practiced satisfactorily by one person. Also, there is practically no mental illness, no mentally disturbed person who will not at one point or another require psychotherapy. Although it is quite true that there will probably never be enough psychiatrists to tend to all those who need help, those para-medical therapists who will be required to practice psychotherapy must have sufficient neurological and psychiatric knowledge, and psychiatric supervision, to be able to make differential diagnoses and to realize when, for example, somatic therapies can be more efficient.

The majority of psychiatrists in the United States are members of the American Psychiatric Association, which has grown from 5,534 members in 1950 to 16,676 in 1971. About 10 per cent of the members of the American Psychiatric Association are psychoanalysts, and there are hardly any psychoanalysts that are not physicians and psychiatrists, since the American Psychoanalytic Society no longer admits applicants who are not physicians and in psychiatric training. Over 60 per cent of the psychiatrists are in private practice, and in 1960 only 1,219 worked exclusively in mental hospitals. The regional distribution of psychiatrists is very uneven. In 1971, the ratio of psychiatrists to 100,000 population ranged from 2.8 in the state of Alabama to 26.6 in the state of New York, and 59.1 in Washington, D. C., the national average being 11.8.

The realization of the plans for decentralization of treatment, for the creation of community mental health centers (1 for 50,000 population), and adequate staffing of mental hospitals will depend on a substantial increase in well-trained psychiatrists, psychologists, and social workers. Studying this particular problem the Joint Commission found that only one tenth of our young people graduate from college. Of those of outstanding intelligence, only about one third finish college and a still smaller percentage enter professional and science graduate programs. Dr. Jack Ewalt, one of the leading psychiatrists in the United States, sadly concluded that "our study suggests that our society does not manifest much respect for the human mind, well or sick."

Presently (as of the end of 1971), there are 108 medical schools in the United States, which graduated 8,974 students in 1971. Of these graduates, about 8 per cent go into psychiatry. The building of new medical schools might help to alleviate some of the shortages in the medical profession in general and in psychiatry in particular, since only about 11,000 students are accepted annually in medical schools out of 25,000 applicants.

The Social Worker:

As members of social agencies caring for the helpless, sick, and destitute, social workers have existed for a long time. The psychiatric social worker was created in 1909 by Adolf Meyer, then professor of psychiatry at the Johns Hopkins University in Baltimore. Meyer was acutely aware of the importance of the environmental factors and surroundings in which his patients lived and became sick. He sent his wife to make visits in the patients' homes, to talk to the relatives, and to take careful case histories. Thus, the original functions of the social worker were to maintain contact among hospital, home, and community and to gather information for an exhaustive social history of the patients. Today, these functions have been widened. Because of the small number of psychiatrists, social workers are indispensable participants in the total therapeutic program for most patients treated in mental hospitals and community mental health clinics. They establish the initial contact with the patient's relatives, gather information from various sources, and assist the patient and his family in the understanding and settling of social and family problems. They enlist the relatives' help, essential in the treatment of the patient. They speak to agencies and prospective employers in preparing the ground for the patient's return to the community, often a difficult and critical step. After a patient's release from the hospital, the social worker frequently remains the most

significant link between the physician and the patient or
his family either by having regular interviews with the
patient or by making occasional home visits. Since today
we are just as much interested in treating as in preventing
mental illness, this is a most important function. (See also
Chapter VII.) According to their ability and training, social
workers conduct group and individual psychotherapy
under the supervision of a psychiatrist.

The social worker's schooling consists of four years of
college and two years of training in a school of social
work, the number of which is rapidly increasing throughout the country. Most social workers have a Masters degree
in Social Work. A few take three additional years of
training leading to a Ph.D. in Social Work.

The Clinical Psychologist:

The psychologist's field of knowledge is man's mental
development and behavior. He is concerned with the
functioning of the senses, such as vision and hearing, with
the process of learning and communication, with intelligence, thinking and memory, and the distortions of these
functions. In today's intricate research activities concerning man, the psychologist works side by side with the
physiologist, the neurophysiologist, the anthropologist,
and the sociologist. A clinical psychologist is the close
associate of psychiatrists and social workers in their
common endeavor to understand and treat the mentally ill.

With respect to understanding mental illness, the
clinical psychologist applies his skills in interviewing and
testing patients. Psychological tests (well selected and

prudently interpreted) can tap regions and dimensions of a patient's personality that are difficult to assess in ordinary psychiatric interviews. To a certain extent, the psychologist can quantify mental abilities, such as intelligence and the degree of organic brain damage. In some instances, the psychologist can help the psychiatrist in understanding a patient's character, motivations, and hidden anxieties, and he can contribute to the formulation of certain diagnoses and treatment plans. Further, he participates in research and in the training of psychiatrists.

Often, the clinical psychologist has a special interest and training in psychotherapy, which he applies in mental hospitals, mental hygiene clinics, and in private practice.

The training of the psychologist consists of four years of college, four years of graduate school in psychology, and a one-year internship in psychology in a recognized mental institution. After having received his Ph.D., the psychologist usually specializes in one of a number of sub-specialties, such as experimental, social, industrial, or clinical psychology.

Diagnostic Aids:

Psychiatric diagnoses are based on careful evaluation of psychopathology. Data from laboratories can specify, suggest, support, or contradict clinical diagnoses, but they cannot establish them. Thus, the examination of the spinal fluid can specify the clinical diagnosis of a chronic brain syndrome by adding that the etiology most likely is a luetic one. An acute brain syndrome may be explained by laboratory findings of a severe anemia, but the presence of an anemia is not synonymous with the diagnosis of a chronic brain syndrome. Psychological tests may demonstrate deterioration of mental faculties and possibly determine that these are organic in nature, but rarely can they specify further.

The psychiatrist uses the laboratories of general medicine and in hospitals routinely examines the composition • of blood, urine, and, if indicated, spinal fluid. He is interested in liver functions, endocrinological studies and X rays of skull, lungs, and spine. Although the practical results of brain wave tests (electroencephalography) are not very rewarding as yet, they may very well become so in the future. Much research is being done in this area and material of potential value is accumulating. The psychiatrist uses the tools of the general practitioner and neurologist, such as the stethoscope, the apparatus to measure blood pressure, the ophthalmoscope, and the reflex hammer. A thorough physical examination is an integral part of a psychiatric one since many serious physical diseases can hide behind psychiatric symptoms.

Of special interest to the psychiatrist are findings from *psychological tests.* There are a great variety of tests used by the psychologist to evaluate intelligence, thinking patterns, emotional balance, and conflicts. The best gauged ones are intelligence tests. Tests that try to elicit content of thought and motivations are subject to considerable interpretation and, thus, lose objectivity. Rorschach's inkblot test may well be the most ingenious and interesting test, with the widest applicability. Although it is difficult to interpret, an experienced psychologist or physician can draw valuable conclusions from it as to the intelligence, character, and psychopathology of his patient.

The extent to which the psychologist, on the basis of test material, can contribute to the understanding of a patient's personality and illness depends on both his ability and the nature of the questions the psychiatrist asks him. If the physician has a clear concept of what psychological tests can and cannot do and if he has an equally precise idea of what he needs to know, he is apt to receive a satisfactory answer. However, if he does not know how to formulate his request for testing, or if he expects the psychologist to help him out with a diagnosis, he ought to be disappointed. In such instances, he is likely to be given information that he could get from clinical interviews or that is unreliable and useless.

Areas in which the psychiatrist can receive constructive help from the psychologist are the following ones: evaluation of intellectual functions, degree of organic brain damage and chances for recovery, a study of the personality, its weakness and strength, and suitability for psychotherapy. If, on the basis of his test results, the psychologist can arrive at a psychiatric diagnosis, he should communicate this to the physician. However, the clinical psychopathology is the decisive factor in the determination of the diagnosis. Discrepancies between clinical impression and psychological tests often occur and are good reasons to further reflect on the case in question.

SUGGESTIONS FOR FURTHER READING

To include an extensive and detailed bibliography would be beyond the scope of this book. Below, the reader will find a partial list of books that will serve as basic references for more detailed studies in the field of psychiatry. The textbooks in particular contain further bibliographies, satisfying the needs of the specialist.

General Psychiatric Literature:

Adler, Alfred, *Theory and Practice of Individual Psychology.* New York, Humanities Press, Inc., 1951.

Alvarez, Walter C., *Minds That Came Back.* New York, J. B. Lippincott Co., 1961.

Arieti, Silvano, ed., *American Handbook of Psychiatry,* 2 vols. New York, Basic Books, Inc., 1959.

Cannon, Walter B., *The Wisdom of the Body,* rev. ed. New York, W. W. Norton & Co., Inc., 1963.

Deutsch, Albert and Fishman, Helen, eds., *The Encyclopedia of Mental Health,* 6 vols. New York, Franklin Watts, Inc., 1963.

Freedman, Alfred M. and Kaplan, Harold, I., *Comprehensive Textbook of Psychiatry.* Baltimore, Williams and Wilkins, 1967.

Freud, Sigmund, *Collected Papers,* edited by Ernest Jones, 5 vols. New York, Basic Books, Inc., 1959.

Gorman, Mike, *Every Other Bed.* Cleveland, The World Publishing Company, 1956.

Jaspers, Karl, *General Psychopathology.* Chicago, University of Chicago Press, 1963.

Jung, Carl G., *Collected Works.* New York, Pantheon Books, 1953-63.

Kallman, Franz J., *Heredity in Health and Mental Disorder.* London, Chapman & Hall, Ltd., 1953.

Kretschmer, Ernst, *Textbook of Medical Psychology.* New York, Oxford University Press, 1934.

Leighton, Alexander H., *et al., Explorations in Social Psychiatry.* New York, Basic Books, Inc., 1957.

Mayer-Gross, W., Slater, Eliot, and Roth, Martin, *Clinical Psychiatry,* 2nd ed. Baltimore, Williams & Wilkins, 1960.

Muncie, W. *Psychobiology and Psychiatry.* St. Louis, C. V. Mosby Co., 1948.

Sheldon, William H.. Stevens, S. S., and Tucker, W. B., *The Varieties of Human Physique.* New York, Harper, 1940.

– – and Stevens, S. S., *The Varieties of Temperament.* New York, Harper, 1942.

Uhr, L. M. and Miller, J. G., eds., *Drugs and Behavior.* New York, John Wiley & Sons, Inc., 1960.

Wiener, Norbert, *Cybernetics,* 2nd ed. New York, John Wiley & Sons, Inc., 1961.

Zilboorg, Gregory, *A History of Medical Psychology.* New York, W. W. Norton & Co., Inc., 1941.

Special Areas of Interest:
Alexander, Franz, *Fundamentals of Psychoanalysis.* New York, Norton, 1948.

– –, *Psychosomatic Medicine.* New York, Norton, 1950.

Bleuler, Eugen, *Dementia Praecox.* New York, International Universities Press, Inc., 1958.

Davidson, H. A., *Forensic Psychiatry.* New York, Ronald Press Company, 1952.

Fromm-Reichmann, F., ed., *Principles of Intensive Psychotherapy.* Chicago, University of Chicago Press, 1950.

– – and Moreno, J. L., eds., *Progress in Psychotherapy.* New York, Grune & Stratton, Inc., 1956.

Horney, Karen, *The Neurotic Personality of Our Time.* New York, Norton, 1937.

– –, *Neurosis and Human Growth.* New York, Norton, 1950.

Jones, Ernest, *The Life and Works of Sigmund Freud,* 3 vols. New York, Basic Books, 1953, 1955, 1957.

Kalinowsky, Lothar B. and Hippius, Hanns, *Pharmacological, Convulsive and Other Somatic Treatments in Psychiatry.* New York, Grune & Stratton, 1969.

Kanner, Leo, *Child Psychiatry,* 3rd ed. Springfield, Ill., C. C. Thomas, 1960.

Kinsey, Alfred, *et al., Sexual Behavior in the Human Female,* Philadelphia, W. B. Saunders & Co., 1953.

– –, *Sexual Behavior in the Human Male.* Philadelphia, W. B. Saunders & Co., 1948.

Lewis, Aubrey, *The State of Psychiatry.* New York, Science House, 1967.

– –, *Inquiries in Psychiatry.* New York, Science House, 1967.

Lorenz, Konrad, *King Solomon's Ring.* New York, T. Y. Crowell, 1952.

– –, *On Aggression.* New York, Bantam Books, 1970.

Masters, William H. and Johnson, Virginia E., *Human Sexual Response.* Boston, Little, Brown, 1966.

– –, – –, *Human Sexual Inadequacy.* Boston, Little, Brown, 1970.

McDougell, William, *An Introduction to Social Psychology.* London, Methuen, 1950.

Monod, Jacques, *Chance and Necessity.* New York, Knopf, 1971.

Pavlov, P., *Conditioned Reflexes*. Gloucester, Mass., Peter Smith, 1960.

Prinzhorn, *Arts of the Mentally Ill*. (German) Berlin, Springer Verlag, 1922.

Skinner, B. F., *Beyond Freedom and Dignity*. New York, Knopf, 1971.

Sherrington, C. S., *The Brain and Its Mechanism*. Cambridge, Cambridge University Press, 1933.

Other Literature of Psychiatric Interest:

Dostoyevsky, Feodor, *Brothers Karamazov*. New York, Grosset & Dunlap, Inc., 1956.

– –, *Crime and Punishment*. New York, Dodd, Mead & Co., 1963.

Huxley, Aldous, *Doors of Perception*. New York, Harper & Row, Publishers, Inc., 1954.

Jaspers, Karl, *Strindberg and Van Gogh*. (Pathography).

Kretschmer, Ernst, *Psychology of Man of Genius*.

– –, *Physique and Character*. London, K. Paul, Trench, Trubner & Co., Ltd.; New York, Harcourt, Brace & Company, Inc., 1925.

Strindberg, August, *The Confession of a Fool*. London, S. Swift, 1912.

– –, *The Inferno*. London, W. Rider & Son, Ltd., 1912.

– –, *Legends*. London, A. Melrose, 1912.

– –, *The Son of a Servant*. New York, G. P. Putnam's Sons, 1913.

Waugh, Evelyn, *Ordeal of Gilbert Pinfold*. Cambridge, Mass., Little, Brown and Company, 1957.

Index

psychoeffective drugs as, 187, 190-197

sedation as, 191-193

tranquilizers, 191-192, 193-194

Manager's disease; *see* Stress

Manic depressive psychosis, 17, 91-103

age factor and, 98, 140, 141

biochemists and, 12

case histories of, 101-103

clinical syndromes of, 92-97

course of, 97-98

etiological considerations of, 91, 99-100

hospitalization and, 141-142

incidence of, 148

prognosis of, 97-98

somatotype and, 32, 92

see also Management, psychiatric

Marplan, 130

Marriage, mental illness and, 227-228

Masturbation, 57

Maudsley, Henry, 3

Mayer-Gross, W., 1, 99, 135, 181

Mayo, J., 210

Medicine, psychosomatic, 65

Meduna, L. J. von, 9, 197

Memory

kinds of, 36

unconscious, 23

Menopause, 44, 59

Mental deficiency, 174

alcoholism and, 178

anatomical findings in, 180

chronic brain syndromes and, 174-181

classification and, 176

cretinism and, 179

definition of, 175

etiological considerations, 179-180

incidence of, 180-181

intelligence level and, 175-176

mongolism and, 179-180

phenylketonuria and, 180

prostitution and, 178

symptomatology and, 176-178

Mental disorders, 148-181

acute brain syndromes in, 149

brain tumors and, 160

causes of, 149

in children, 153

comments on, 149-152

definition of, 149, 152

endocrine diseases and, 157-158

examples of, 149

head injuries and, 158-160

infectious diseases and, 152-154

intoxication and, 154-157

introduction to, 148-149

lesions and, 153

metabolic diseases and, 157-158

alcoholism and; *see* Alcoholism

causes of, 4

chronic brain syndromes in, 82

brain tumor and, 169-171

case histories of, 163-166, 169-171

causes of, 149

comments on, 148-152, 160-161

definition of, 149, 160

encephalitis and, 82

examples of, 149-150

idiopathic epilepsy and, 171-174

infectious diseases and, 161-166

intoxications and, 166-167

mental deficiency and, 174-181

old age and, 167-169

syphilis and, 163-166

classification of, 4, 13

concepts of, 14-52

cultural patterns and, 6

definitions of, 14-18

delusions in, 23

diagnosis of, 46-50

emotional experience and, 6

environment and, 6, 37-40

etiology of, 24-28, 43-46, 54, 148-181

explanation of, 40-42

genetics and, 28-30

hallucinations in, 23, 25-26, 113-114